You Are What You Digest *by* Christine Tara Peterson

YOU ARE WHAT YOU DIGEST

Christine Tara Peterson
Ph.D., A.H.P., R.Y.T.

Printed, Published & Distributed by

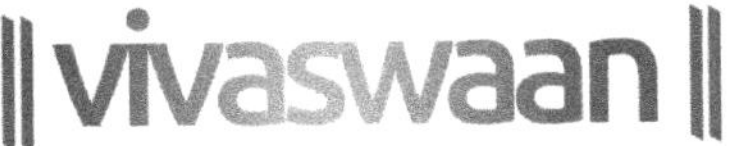

www.vivaswaan.com

Designed & published by VIVASWAAN
Formerly *Vedic Wisdom Press*
Now wholly owned subsidiary of
Vedic Management Group LLC, Sheridan (WY) USA.
www.vivaswaan.com

ISBN:
First Impression
10 9 8 7 6 5 4 3 2 1

Printed in:
India by *Thomson Press Limited*
Europe by *Lego Press*
USA by *Ingram Publications*

Table of Contents

Part 1
How the Microbiome Works

The idiom "you are what you eat" has been modified for the title of this book to *"You Are What You Digest" and absorb*. We must amend these statements since they are true yet may not be as precise as they once were due to intensive research on the gut microbiota over the past two decades.

Introduction
Health Empowerment
Through Information

An Overview

Welcome to a fascinating voyage through the world of microbes that live inside of you. This book is divided into three sections and serves primarily as an introduction to the gut microbiome (Part 1). Considerable effort was made to describe the gut microbiome in understandable terms, minimizing the use of scientific jargon and presenting complex scientific concepts in plain language. Similarly, our knowledge of gut microbiomes dictates the far reach of our gut microbes to systems operating outside of the gut.

In Part 2 of the book, we examine the relationship between several chronic diseases that have been on the rise in human populations over the past few decades and the gut microbiome. Attempts were made to describe these diseases in detail without using confusing terminology so that readers could more fully understand and appreciate the influence of gut microorganisms on such a wide range of diseases. A fundamental theme of the book relates to the dichotomy of our gut microbiome as both a powerful ally in maintaining excellent health and a mediator of disease. The path upon which our gut microbiome places us is largely determined by our own actions and choices, particularly with regards to our dietary habits.

Finally, Part 3 details dietary and lifestyle considerations for a healthy gut microbiome. Later chapters present an introduction to Ayurveda, an ancient and powerful traditional system of medicine from India. Given the complexities of Ayurvedic medicine, it became apparent that readers would benefit from receiving the necessary context and background information to fully appreciate and comprehend the inherent logic of this therapeutic modality. The solution to this dilemma necessitated a comprehensive explanation of the gut microbiome (Part 1). This topic may be complex, but it is essential for understanding the far-reaching health benefits that can be attained through the daily application of Ayurvedic principles.

Maintaining good health in the information age.

A multitude of books address health, diet, and well-being. The abundance of information and variety of perspectives reflect the complexity of nutrition and health as well as the widespread desire of people around the world to increase their knowledge of how to live a healthy and meaningful life. The internet era has increased our cognizance of the stories of human illness told by afflicted individuals. Today, environmental factors that promote health and cause disease are more widely recognized. We are all more motivated to take personal responsibility for our health, regardless of whether our desire to learn more is motivated by a dread of disease and the difficulties associated with illness or by a desire to optimize our own health and well-being.

As a society, we now have greater access to information regarding the diseases that affect many millions of people worldwide, including millions of Americans. Chronic illness has a significant impact on quality of life, and those who endure it require solutions. Typically, these solutions prove more elusive than anticipated, and we discover that we need assistance sifting through the copious and potentially contradictory information provided by an increasing number of sources.

Today, new scientific discoveries are being made at an unprecedented rate. This is facilitated by technological advancements that have accelerated the rate of new discoveries that challenge our worldview and perception of reality. This is true of all scientific fields, but especially those pertaining to human health. As a result of numerous victories and incremental advances, our understanding of the fundamental human systems and subsystems that malfunction in the context of disease has significantly expanded. The information gathered regarding the factors that promote healthful aging is also crucial. These developments have illustrated the diversity and complexity of both health and disease.

It's all Greek to me.

Frequently, it becomes necessary to translate scientific terminology and the conceptual frameworks underlying new scientific discoveries. This translation need not be exhaustive, but it should use terminology that facilitates comprehension of new ideas and findings. The value of basic knowledge of health-related topics is growing. An increasing number of natural products on the market today claim to hold the key to restoring health. If consumers are to make intelligent use of natural remedies, they must be aware of the limitations and precautions associated with them.

This book is intended to provide insightful, fundamental information about natural remedies. These suggestions are intended to strengthen your discernment, not replace your physician's advice. Natural remedies and traditional health practices are most effective when used under the supervision of a qualified health practitioner.

The primary impediment to self-education on health-related topics is the extensive use of jargon and complex biological and scientific details that obscure the fundamental message, which is frequently easy to understand. This book strives to provide the most reliable, empirically-based scientific facts in a language that is accessible to nearly everyone. Some complex and even abstract concepts and ideas are discussed. Efforts were made to elucidate terms and explain concepts in the most straightforward manner possible so that readers appreciate the enthusiasm and optimism that recent discoveries have inspired. This information is provided with the intention that it will better equip readers to understand their healthcare options and safeguard them against low-quality products.

People are becoming more aware that the healthcare system does not always provide the answers they seek, particularly in the context of chronic conditions. In addition, health insurance providers frequently fall short in providing the coverage required to fully recover. This is especially true for those who choose natural, non-pharmaceutical options for chronic illness. Many pharmaceutical drugs are focused on treating symptoms, and discerning customers today are cognizant of the negative effects of prolonged drug use. As a consequence of these and other discoveries, the demand for pharmacological complements and alternatives has increased.

The importance of diet and lifestyle.

Despite its best intentions, easily accessible health information often oversimplifies health and disease, leaves readers confused, or presents only one side of the story. In order to empower readers with information on optimal health, the book focuses primarily on background information covering the gut microbiome as well as dietary and lifestyle recommendations that are both easy to understand and apply.

The effect of a Western diet on human health is one example that will be thoroughly discussed in this book. A western diet is characterized by high-calorie, high-fat, highly-processed-ingredient, high-refined-sugar, and often nutrient-deficient meals. Given the available scientific evidence, it is reasonable to assert that the western diet directly contributes to the type 2 diabetes and obesity epidemics in both developed and developing nations. Although we cannot confirm this with certainty at this time, there may also be strong associations with other chronic disorders.

In this volume, we explore topics that have been the subject of extensive independent scientific research.

There is evidence presented to help guide lifestyle and dietary choices. We investigate several topics in which comprehensive understanding is still deficient. This information also serves as a caution to readers to be skeptical of health-promoting claims made by commercial products for which there is a lack of solid scientific evidence.

This book provides a novel examination of common gut-related conditions. A list of maladies whose prevalence has increased dramatically over the past few decades is given special consideration. Rather than relying solely on genetics to explain these patterns, we must investigate our diet, way of life, and long-term exposure to environmental factors that promote the chronic diseases of our time. These diseases are not only preventable but frequently treatable as well.

Our gut bacteria are contradictory.

Trillions of bacteria inhabit the human body and impact our health. The human microbiota is the collective name for these microbial communities, which have a substantial impact on human health that may be either beneficial or detrimental. The first section of the book looks at how our nutrition and immune system interact with the bacteria that live in our small and large intestines to affect our health. The sum total of genes found in the bacteria that live in our guts is referred to as the gut microbiome. The community or collection of bacteria that lives in our gut is referred to as the gut microbiota. We will explore how the gut microbiota transforms the food we eat into substances that can maintain or enhance our health through its many activities. Additionally, we will discover how and why eating a poor diet makes people sick. We will also learn how the gut microbiota affects our immune system's functioning in order to change how it can either prevent or worsen disease.

The gut microbiota's dual role as one of our most powerful allies and dangerous potential foes suggests that we are best served by taking proactive measures to keep our tiny counterparts as friends. The reader will learn from this book how to develop and maintain a lifelong, mutually beneficial connection with our bacteria. The idiom "you are what you eat" has been modified for the title of this book to *"You Are What You Digest" and absorb*. This proverb undoubtedly contains wisdom, which is one of the reasons it has endured throughout time. We must amend these statements since they are true yet not as precise as they once were due to intensive research on the gut microbiota over the past two decades. We will explore why this distinction is critical and why the modification that *"you are what you digest and absorb"* is more correct.

In the past two decades, the gut microbiota has received considerable attention as one of the important environmental factors that influence disease. Our current understanding of the gut microbiota emphasizes its significance for optimal gut function and how dysbiosis, a condition in which the microbiota is out of balance, can result in disease. The second chapter will provide a more comprehensive definition of the term dysbiosis. Diet is believed to be the most influential variable affecting the equilibrium or imbalance of the intestinal microbiota. In this sense, consuming nutritious foods that promote a healthy intestinal flora may be the best way to maintain outstanding health and vitality throughout your life.

Our microbiome determines the health benefits of the food we eat. A portion of the food we consume is chemically altered or converted by gut microbes, which increases the bioactivity of specific nutrients and the bioavailability of nutrients that are not readily assimilated. Although this is significant, there is much more to the story, as it is likely that some microorganisms are exceptionally adept at a biochemistry that generates compounds with drug-like, health-promoting properties.

Let's get to it.

Before humans existed, bacterial communities made an agreement with their primordial animal hosts. Microbes offered its host greater energy and nutrient yield from their diet in exchange for improved accommodations and sustenance. This advantage may have motivated the establishment of a close association with the immune system, a second important element of the agreement. Beginning with the Cambrian explosion, primitive mammals developed the capacity to tolerate microbes over a period of more than 500 million years. It is conceivable that over time, immune systems have treated bacteria with the ability to increase the amount of energy derived from food while also improving the fitness of their hosts more favorably. According to this theory, primitive immune systems may have also played a long-term role in the accord with bacterial inhabitants that led to the extremely complex interaction between humans and bacteria that we observe today; however, this has only recently been recognized. The discovery that communication between the gut microbiota and the immune system is bidirectional and that bacteria not only respond to the immune system but also provide it instructions to enable protection against infections and even the elimination of tumors is perhaps the most astounding.

Consequently, the close, interdependent relationship we have with our resident microbes is essential to our health, which is why it is so important to maintain the harmony it provides. Mutualism is the term used to characterize cooperative interactions between two or more organisms in which both individuals benefit from the relationship. In contrast to pathogenic and parasitic partnerships, this partnership does not injure or impede the fitness of one or more of its members.

Our understanding of how the gut microbiota impacts our health and how it may cause disease when it becomes unbalanced as a result of consuming the wrong foods is constantly expanding. Contrary to appearances, the bacteria in our intestines are not acting in rebellion; rather, they are simply surviving in the environments they occupy while receiving the fundamental nutrients they require. The choice of the foods that we feed our intestinal flora is up to us. Diet is the most effective way to directly influence whether the microorganisms in your intestines are working for or against you. For example, some foods, such as charred meat, are unhealthy due to the ability of intestinal microbes to convert nutritional components into toxic and even mutagenic molecules. It is plausible that our gut microorganisms ultimately determine whether the food we consume is healthy or unhealthy. Surprisingly, despite increased knowledge and advanced scientific research, we continue to acknowledge that our mothers were correct in advising us to eat our vegetables and limit our intake of desserts and junk food.

The rise of many illnesses.

In the second section of this book, we will examine a number of gut-related conditions whose prevalence has increased significantly in both industrialized and developing nations. Many of us are aware of how our dietary choices impact our health. In the past, it was believed that the connection between food and health resulted from the function of our digestive system, which assimilated the nutrients we ate so that they could directly enter the bloodstream and provide energy to our tissues.

The importance of the gastrointestinal microbiota in the relationship between diet and health was only recently recognized. This discovery has sparked a new revolution in the biomedical sciences, forcing us to reconsider what we previously believed about human health and disease. The significance of the study of the human microbiome has made it increasingly apparent that this information must be shared with the general public. As more clinical disorders are associated with the actions of gut flora, the importance of this endeavor will grow.

By reading this book, you will better understand gut-related information provided to you by your physician and health practitioners and hopefully make even more informed health choices. Second, and likely more substantially, your dietary choices have the greatest impact on your microbiome status. In this regard, you, the reader, will have greater knowledge and ability to help preserve a healthy microbiome.

The considerable association between environmental factors, such as our eating patterns, and chronic diseases that have become more prevalent in recent years demonstrates that we all have the ability to alter our own health. Diet, particularly long-term dietary patterns, has a substantial impact on the bacterial populations in our intestines and, consequently, on our health. As we shall see, the influence of gastrointestinal microorganisms extends beyond the gut and digestive health to impact the immune system of the entire body. In this way, gut microbes influence not only the risk of developing type 2 diabetes (Chapter 9) or colon cancer (Chapter 10), but also affect distant organ systems such as the brain (Chapter 11).

Your health will change if your microbiota changes.

In the third section of the book, we will examine a variety of natural remedies that can restore healthy levels of intestinal flora. Utilizing natural constituents such as dietary fibers, medicinal herbs, and chemical compounds found in fruits and vegetables are the most effective methods for altering the composition of gut microbiota. Both stand-alone and supplementary interventions that target the gut microbiota to restore health hold great promise.

Most clinicians are beginning to educate themselves on the therapeutic potential of a healthy intestinal flora. After years of attentively observing their patients, many gastroenterologists have developed an intuition that has prepared them for the possibility of using microbial-based treatments in the future. A growing number of alternative and integrative medicine physicians are establishing offices in response to the increasing demand for healthcare that incorporates both conventional and traditional (natural) approaches to human health. As the trajectory of science and medicine clearly indicates, it is only a matter of time before a new era of therapeutic modulation of gut microbiomes dawns.

While the prospect of a new paradigm in disease treatment is encouraging, it is essential to remember that disease prevention is always preferable to disease treatment. Our hectic schedules and ambitions frequently prevent us from acting in the best interest of our health. We frequently indulge in vices, such as eating our favored unhealthy foods, due to our daily stressors. Consequently, embracing our own health is a mental and physical challenge. Ultimately, the first step in assuming personal responsibility for our health is gaining the ability to alter our behaviors.

Dietary modification is one of the most difficult challenges we will face on our health journey. Recognizing the scope of challenge is a crucial aspect of any self-inventory you may desire to conduct. Such introspection will reveal whether you can accomplish your health objectives on your own or if you require professional assistance, such as from a psychologist, physician, herbalist, nutritionist, or health coach, to help you create or maintain a healthy diet and lifestyle.

By exploring this book, you will have taken a significant step toward educating yourself about a fascinating subject as well as simple solutions and ideas that you likely never considered significant. Due to the scope of this volume, it is exceedingly difficult to do justice to many of the covered topics and to describe the inner workings of the human body in great detail. This work's presentational style will assist you in locating the most pertinent information and distinguishing between biased and objective material. In some instances, the presentations may inspire further reading. Wikipedia, which typically provides accurate and thorough explanations as well as relevant reading recommendations in the field of science, and PubMed from the National Institutes of Health should be consulted frequently when concepts are unclear.

Let us embark on an exciting quest for better health by learning about our unseen microbial companions, what drives them, how they behave, and how this knowledge is the key to a long and healthy life. Let us all strive to make responsible, intelligent health decisions for ourselves and our families. While it takes dedication and self-discipline to make the necessary lifestyle changes for long-term health, the benefits are well worth the effort.

While there is currently nothing that can be done about the genetic hand you have been dealt, you have the ability to alter your nutrition and microbiome in order to counteract the effects of the majority of mutations that make you susceptible to disease. The discovery of the microbiome and epigenome show that we are not slaves to our genes but have great power in altering our health.

Chapter 1. Trends in Recent Decades Regarding Disease

Realizing our desires, but at what cost?

We frequently compare ourselves, our behaviors, our cultural norms, our ideals, and our social standing to those of previous generations. While some aspects of our lives have improved, others appear to be worse than those of our parents and ancestors. People in many countries may attest to positive change because they are wealthier and more educated than their parents. This is the simple dream and aspiration of every parent: to give their offspring a better existence. The desire for their children's health and happiness is among the most essential of these objectives. The majority of parents pursue this objective primarily by attempting to increase their financial security.

Herein lies a critical paradox: Are we realizing this dream? Are we healthier than our ancestors? The instinctive response would be yes, of course we are. Over the past several generations, advances in technology, medical procedures, access to health care, and drug discovery have significantly increased the human lifespan. When we do become ill, we are reassured that medical science has advanced so significantly that our physicians will have the most effective remedies to restore our health. This may be true, but it does not adequately resolve the query, "Are we now healthier?" The trends are contradictory, but it is undeniable that the incidence of numerous diseases that affect millions of people has increased in developed countries, suggesting that we are sicker than our ancestors in many respects.

In the past few decades, the landscape of gastrointestinal disorders has changed dramatically. Peanut allergies, gluten intolerance, inflammatory bowel disease (IBD), and irritable bowel syndrome (IBS) were undoubtedly unfamiliar to our parents. As adolescents, we all had classmates who were overweight or even obese, but they were less common than they are today. When disease incidence increases dramatically over a few decades, human genetics cannot completely explain the underlying causes. This is due to the fact that genetic changes (evolution) do not occur on such brief time intervals. On the other hand, it does not rule out the possibility that pre-existing mutations in the population are crucial disease susceptibility factors. Therefore, we must investigate environmental factors to fill in the gaps. How do environmental factors like our diet interact with our genetic make-up to determine our susceptibility to disease?

Humans are ill and growing sicker.

The plain summary of our health status in the 21st century is that we are more likely than previous generations to develop disease during our lifetimes, and that by extending our lifespans, we increase this likelihood even further. The causes of our deteriorating health are complex and multifaceted. But the reality is that each of us has a straightforward decision to make. Accept that we may become the victim of a serious disease during our lifetimes and trust that medical science will come to the rescue, or pursue a more radical option that involves recognizing that the trends in human health indicate that we must assume a greater level of personal responsibility for our health if we wish to avoid being a part of the health care crisis.

Getting ill impacts your finances.

Large pharmaceutical corporations have concluded that preventative medicine is not economically viable for a variety of reasons, including a fundamental dearth of demand. Therefore, the practice of preventative medicine falls solely on you or non-mainstream clinicians, who are likely not covered by your health insurance. Your family doctor may advise you to lose weight or reduce the amount of sodium you add to your diet. If your blood pressure is critically excessive, your doctor may decide to prescribe a blood pressure-lowering medication. Taking your doctor's advice may be the most judicious decision of your life, but this should not be the conclusion of your story, but rather the beginning of a new chapter.

Serious illness may not only endanger your life, but also your financial security. As debilitating to your family's stability as the disease itself can be, soaring health care costs and more restricted health care coverage. Whether your motivation to take control of your health stems from a desire to protect your family's hard-earned savings, college and retirement funds or a strong desire to live a long and healthy life, the best available insurance policy is to simply remain healthy.

Weighing your priorities.

When asked what astonished him most about humanity, His Holiness the Dalai Lama replied, "Man. Because he sacrifices his health in order to make money. Then he sacrifices money to recuperate his health. Then, he is so anxious about the future that he does not enjoy the present; as a result, he does not live in the present or the future; he lives as if he will never die, and he dies having never truly lived." These wise words should cause each of us to pause and reflect on their applicability to our own lives.

Take a moment to list the five most important items in your existence. Once you have completed this, return to the list and determine how many of the items are directly or indirectly dependent on your health and ability to live an active existence. Possibly all or the majority of the enumerated values depend on your health and wellbeing. We are all adept at putting first things first, balancing obligations to our family, colleagues, and careers. It is much more difficult to prioritize preventative measures for something that may never occur or will not be a problem for 20 years. This is the lamentable reality of health and disease; we simply do not know our fate and, consequently, how much of our valuable time we should devote to our health. As we will see in the following section, the trends in disease incidence make it apparent that each of us must give greater attention to our health if we wish to avoid becoming a statistic. Ultimately, it comes down to establishing your priorities: you can pay now by modifying your lifestyle, or you can pay later by experiencing the agony and anguish that accompany a health crisis.

The evolution of our demand for fast food.

In just two generations, the number of families with two working parents has increased dramatically. The number of hours we spend working each week is increasing, and the time we have to unwind and appreciate the fruits of our labor appears to be decreasing. Working 40, 50, or even 60 hours per week leaves parents with little time or energy for grocery shopping, let alone purchasing foods that require time and effort to prepare. Historically, as more women entered the workforce in the 1950s and 1960s, a demand arose for family-friendly dishes that could be prepared and consumed swiftly. This demand had a direct impact on the number of fast-food options that were made available to us. Since then, this upward trend in demand has persisted unabatedly.

It is essential to recognize that the food industry is a massive enterprise. According to Business Review USA, the combined sales of the top 10 food and beverage manufacturers exceeded $214 billion in 2014. These industry titans have responded to our demand for rapid and appetizing food by providing an unprecedented variety of processed foods and beverages that are designed to taste better than the majority of the natural whole foods we consume. We have gradually developed a craving for these high-fat, high-sugar, high-calorie, low-nutrient foods. The purpose here is not to assign culpability to the consumer or the manufacturer of such foods, but rather to acknowledge this reality and recognize its impact on our health and wellbeing.

In a typical grocery store, one or, on rare occasions, two aisles are devoted to fresh produce and whole foods, while the remaining aisles are filled with processed foods, such as canned goods, packaged foods, prepackaged meals, soft beverages, and frozen foods. Many of these items are challenging to objectively classify as foods. The increasing popularity of fast-food restaurants has introduced our society to foods that are generally high in fat and low in nutritional value. According to franchisehelp.com, there are over two hundred thousand fast food restaurants in the United States that serve fifty million consumers daily

Slowly but certainly, we have become accustomed to this way of life, and as expected, we have devised justifications for the shortcuts we choose to take. Is this simply a consequence of progress? Perhaps, but as we become increasingly aware of the repercussions of our affluent modern lifestyle, we must reconsider the price we pay for expediency. Examining the trends in disease incidence, particularly those that have increased to an alarming degree over the past few decades, prompts scientists, medical physicians, and the general public to inquire, "What is causing these increases?" The brief answer is that there is no single cause. However, overwhelming evidence supports the notion that our recently adopted diet is a significant factor.

Changing what we demand

As of March 2016, it was estimated that there are 7.4 billion persons on earth. The United Nations estimates that the global population will reach over 9 billion by 2050 and 11.2 billion by 2100. Overpopulation may be the single greatest hazard to the survival of our species. There are numerous reasons for this, but if we investigate the problem inherent in nourishing and providing clean potable water for 7.4 billion people, we can gain a better understanding of why the foods we consume today do not nourish and sustain our health. The increased demand for food has had a profound effect on global agricultural practices and the varieties of crops and livestock that are raised.

Large, highly mechanized farms have largely supplanted small family farms. To increase crop yields and efficacy, extensive farmland is monoculture (one crop). This practice depletes vital soil nutrients over time, reducing crop yields and increasing plant susceptibility to parasites. Farmers are compelled to use increasing amounts of herbicides, pesticides, and fertilizers to maximize crop yields.

To optimize profits per acre, new genetic variants of crops have been developed to increase the size and aesthetic qualities of fruits and vegetables. The capacity of the family farmer to survive in an era of diminishing profits requires these producers to adopt these practices. The question is to what extent these practices deprive us of the nutrients that fresh produce provides. There have been comparisons between conventionally and organically raised crops. Surprisingly, none of these 55 studies demonstrated that the nutrient content of organic produce was superior to that of conventionally grown produce.

A meta-analysis of these studies concluded that few were conducted with appropriate controls or thoroughness and therefore could not be used for comparisons, but the remaining studies did not reveal any significant differences. Given the significance of the concerns raised by these studies, it is a disgrace that definitive answers are not yet available. However, one undeniable advantage of organic produce is that it is free of herbicides and pesticides, for which there is ample evidence of their detrimental effects on human physiology. Similarly, conventionally raised livestock are treated with antibiotics and growth hormones, whereas organically raised livestock are not. In chapters 7 and 9, we will delve deeply into the effects of antibiotics and how they affect allergy and obesity.

Farmers and food producers, like any other corporation, will supply the market with what is profitable and in demand. If consumers request organic, unprocessed foods, suppliers will respond accordingly. Suppliers will continue to provide inexpensive, convenient, high-calorie, low-nutrient foods if we continue to consume them. We are beginning to observe a trend toward a demand for healthy foods in the most unlikely of settings: fast food restaurants, which continue to offer burgers and fries but also increasingly offer healthier options. This transformation is not an act of charity; rather, it is a response to consumer demand that enables fast food chains to maintain high profits and returns to investors. This plainly demonstrates the influence we have as consumers to effect positive change through our demand.

Epidemic diseases in the 21st century.

The obesity epidemic. Obesity, among the maladies exhibiting epidemic growth in recent decades, is perhaps the most significant and is directly linked to dietary behavior changes. According to the CDC, adult obesity in the United States has more than doubled from 1980 to 2010 (from 14% to 35%), with projections that 42% of the population will be obese by 2030. Even more alarming is the increase in adolescent adiposity that has been observed. According to bariatric–surgery-source.com, between 1963 and 1970, boys and girls between the ages of

6 and 19 had an obesity rate of just over 3.5 percent. These rates began to rise at an alarming rate in the early 1980s, and by 2008, boys between the ages of 6 and 11 showed the greatest increase, reaching 15 to 20 percent. According to The American Journal of Clinical Nutrition, the consumption of high fructose corn syrup in the United States increased significantly commencing in the mid-1970s, when the average consumption was close to 0 grams per day. By the turn of the century in 2000, daily consumption had increased to nearly 80 grams on average. While the United States and Mexico have the highest obesity rates, these trends are not unique to these nations; many others, including those with a historically low prevalence of obesity such as Korea, are experiencing increases at comparable rates.

Obesity and its related conditions. Obesity contributes to the development of a wide range of life-threatening and life-shortening diseases, including type 2 diabetes, coronary heart disease, non-alcoholic fatty liver disease, and others. Incidence rates for type 2 diabetes were 1% in 1958 and progressively increased to 3% by 1994, according to data compiled by Medscape.com. In 2006, this affected more than 6% of the U.S. population, or approximately 19 million people. Again, the high-fat and high-sugar Western diet is cited as a significant factor in the observed trends. Surprisingly, the incidence of cardiovascular disease, which includes coronary heart disease, stroke, and other heart diseases, has increased only marginally from 1997 to 2011, while the mortality rate attributable to these conditions has plummeted over the same time period due to advances in detection and treatment.

Autism spectrum disorders (ASD). Autism spectrum disorder is one of the most alarming trends in severe diseases today. According to the CDC, the incidence of ASD increased from 4.2 per 1,000 children in 1996 to 15.5 per 1,000 children in 2010. Other sources indicate both a higher frequency and a faster rate of growth. Autism spectrum disorder is considered a neurodevelopmental disorder and is believed to be the consequence of excessive neuronal development in some brain regions and insufficient neuronal development in others. These observations are consistent with the characteristics of individuals with ASD, who may exhibit varying degrees of behavioral and social difficulties, as well as high cognitive abilities in other domains, such as memory and mathematics.

It is debatable whether the incidence of autism spectrum disorder (ASD) is genuinely on the rise or whether the increased frequency is due to increased awareness and more thorough screening, resulting in an increase in disease diagnosis. Whether ASD can be induced in children with ostensibly normal development as a consequence of vaccinations or other immune disruptions is a subject of increasing controversy. In Chapter 11, we will examine these gut-brain concerns and others.

Additionally, autoimmune diseases are on the rise in the population. Sjogren's syndrome, thyroid disease, scleroderma, Myasthenia gravis, rheumatoid arthritis, and multiple sclerosis disproportionately affect women. This is because genetic and environmental triggers interact with endocrine sex hormones, resulting in the onset of autoimmune disorders. According to the American Autoimmune Related Disease Association (AARDA), approximately 50 million Americans are affected by autoimmune disease.

In addition to their prevalence, individuals with autoimmune disorders frequently exhibit nonspecific symptoms dominated by fatigue. Sixty percent of individuals with an autoimmune disease report that fatigue is the most debilitating symptom, preventing them from performing tasks that the rest of us take for granted. Sadly, 90% of afflicted individuals reported discussing fatigue with their doctor, but 60% of those individuals did not obtain a prescription or treatment recommendation. While generalized fatigue can be caused by a variety of factors, it is frequently misdiagnosed as a sign of depression, thereby denying patients access to appropriate treatment options or, worse, prescribing them antidepressant medication unnecessarily.

The prevalence of allergies is on the rise. From 1998-2000 to 2004-2006, the number of individuals under the age of 18 discharged from hospitals with a diagnosis of food allergy nearly quadrupled, according to a CDC report. Two to three times more likely to develop asthma, eczema, or respiratory allergy were children diagnosed with food allergy before the age of 18. These findings are consistent with experimental evidence linking food allergy to more widespread immune tolerance alterations.

Celiac disease. Gluten intolerance is an example of a clinical condition that has not been recognized by the majority of the population. Gluten-free diets are viewed by many as yet another dietary novelty with no clinical basis. The vast majority of clinicians and individuals with gluten intolerance are aware that this is not the case. Celiac disease, a significant gastrointestinal disorder that is considered an autoimmune disease, is caused by gluten intolerance. According to the Celiac Disease Foundation, 1 in 100 persons worldwide have celiac disease. Even more alarming are estimates that 2.5 million Americans remain undiagnosed and, as a result, are at risk for developing additional complications due to immune abnormalities and atrophy due to impaired assimilation of essential nutrients in the small intestine.

The frustration of not belonging

A growing number of patients with gastro-intestinal, autoimmune, and allergic conditions initially present with subclinical symptoms and therefore do not fit neatly into predefined disease and treatment protocols. This is exemplified by the increasing number of people who suffer from intestinal permeability, a condition commonly referred to as "leaky gut syndrome." This dysfunction may be a common predisposing factor for a significant number of diseases that have become epidemic in recent times. In Chapter 8, we will revisit the topic of leaky gut as a common underlying condition, emphasizing the critical significance of enhanced diagnosis and treatment of leaky gut patients.

There are no reliable estimates of the total number of individuals who experience occasional constipation or diarrhea, low energy, poor sleep, fatigue, and other subclinical symptoms. After all, who doesn't experience these issues occasionally? The problem is that we have come to regard these situations as normal. Symptoms that occur once or twice a year may gradually become more frequent, occurring four to five times a year and then two to three times a month, with each occurrence being accepted as "normal." We are susceptible to rationalizing these vague but important warning signs, possibly because we do not feel qualified to solve them and because they do not properly constitute being unwell, so we do not seek assistance as we would for other, more obvious illnesses.

Numerous individuals with chronic digestive problems live their lives in this manner. At the very least, living with these issues reduces our quality of life, and at worst, disregarding the early warning signs may put us at risk for developing a life-threatening illness. By educating yourself about these benign symptoms, monitoring their occurrence, and identifying the behaviors that appear to trigger them, you become a better patient for your physician. Frequently, the doctor's ability to recognize the complications of early warning signs depends on the information you provide.

The Path to Health

If concerns become significant, it is recommended to keep a record of your diet or exposures to other environmental factors, as well as the emergence of subtle abnormalities or symptoms. This straightforward advice could help you receive an accurate diagnosis early on, thereby preventing unnecessary suffering and distress associated with such symptoms. While doctors are increasingly recognizing the cause-and-effect relationships of these symptoms, they remain outside of mainstream diagnoses and patients are more likely to be misdiagnosed or told "nothing is wrong with you," leaving you to wonder if your symptoms are "all in your head."

We will focus specifically on these chronic diseases because they all represent instances in which human genetics, nutrition, and intestinal microbiota interact as disease-causing factors. While there is currently nothing that can be done about the genetic hand you have been dealt, you have the ability to alter your nutrition and microbiome in order to counteract the effects of the majority of mutations that make you susceptible to disease. The discovery of the microbiome and epigenome (modifications to DNA that alter expression of proteins) show that we are not slaves to our genes but have great power in altering our health. In the following chapter, we will investigate the interaction between genes and mutations and the environment.

We should all consider ourselves exceedingly privileged to have a second chance for health in the context of many diseases as the errors of the past can be rectified by merely altering our behaviors, habits and routines.

Chapter 2
It's All in Your Genes...Or Is It?

Genetics and disease susceptibility: more than 3 billion base pairs.

Just like society, biomedical research follows trends and focuses on fashionable topics. What is in fashion is generally justified but not necessarily correct or holding the secrets to disease we think. In science, trends have a propensity to generate dogma, which, once established, can be difficult to overturn. Thankfully, even though they are susceptible to following trends, scientists require evidence for their continued belief in prevailing dogma. In the absence of such evidence, scientists immediately shift their focus to a new and enhanced hypothesis. One such trend in the biological sciences was the notion that human genetics accounted for the majority of diseases. In the end, research findings disproved this view, necessitating a reevaluation of how we perceive disease.

With the more widespread capacity to sequence genes and examine genetic variations in human populations, we have a clearer understanding that genetics play a significant role in disease incidence, but that genetics are not the only factor. The premise of the age-old nature versus nurture debate seems to urge individuals to adopt sides. In reality, we have learned that human disease is not an either-or situation. Your genetic makeup interacts with a vast array of environmental factors to determine your individual susceptibility to disease.

Fitbit and other personal monitoring devices are likely to increase in utility, allowing individuals to collect vast quantities of data pertaining to numerous aspects of our daily activities and physiological responses to them. When this information is combined with your genetic information, future clinicians may be significantly better able to identify disease, its causes, and most importantly, the optimal course of treatment to make you well again.

Human genome sequencing

The complete DNA sequence present in a cell is referred to as its genome. The typical bacterial genome consists of a single circular chromosome with approximately 3 million base pairs. In comparison, the human genome consists of over 3 billion base pairs of DNA distributed across 23 pairs of chromosomes. At the time of your conception, a sperm cell containing 23 unpaired chromosomes fertilized an egg containing 23 unpaired chromosomes from your mother. Whether or not that sperm cell contained an X or Y sex chromosome determined your gender. Fertilization ensures that, with the exception of specialized cells called gametes (eggs and sperm), each cell in your body contains 23 pairs of chromosomes.

The number of genes encoding proteins in the human genome is still actively debated and range from 20,000-25,000. Many were dismayed by the fact that the human genome encoded a relatively small number of genes, given the relative sophistication of our species. In the end, we are aware of single-celled bacteria that encode 8,000 to 9,000 protein-coding genes. How is it that humans encode only two to three times as many genes as a basic bacterium? This question is beyond the scope of this volume, but suffice it to say that gene count is not the greatest indicator of intelligence. A distinct and more appropriate viewpoint is to marvel at how much the human species can accomplish with so few genes.

Technological advancements allow us to ascertain the nucleotide sequence of our genome with increased efficiency and drastically decreased costs. As the cost of sequencing the human genome continues to decline, it may become commonplace for clinicians to request that your genome be sequenced to aid in disease diagnosis. Since the publication of the first two human genomes in

2003, thousands of additional genomes have been sequenced. It is difficult to estimate the exact number because many are determined by private companies that are unlikely to disclose their data. It is likely that more than 10,000,000 human genomes have been sequenced, and this figure is projected to rise dramatically over the next decade.

To date, human genome sequencing has been performed primarily as part of concentrated efforts to comprehend the frequency of mutations associated with specific diseases, but it is not yet applicable to the average person who visits their doctor for an annual checkup. The sequencing of the human genome is being actively pursued in the field of cancer. The early successes of this form of data suggest that this strategy will be expanded. Scientists from around the globe are analyzing tumor samples for mutations and genetic abnormalities. According to the findings of these studies, malignancies are typically highly heterogeneous and mutate at a rapid rate. This information was crucial in determining the most effective protocols for eradicating the tumor and is a prime example of how medicine is increasingly shifting toward personalized approaches.

By analyzing the types of mutations present in any type of tumor, such as breast cancer, oncologists are able to rapidly determine the likely efficacy of one treatment over another. Since not all breast tumors are identical, neither should their treatment fall under a single, predetermined procedure. The heterogeneity of mutations within a single tumor has also contributed to our understanding of why some chemotherapeutic treatments are only partially effective and why drug resistance develops. More detail will be provided in Chapter 11. Oncologists must be devoted scholars of the academic literature and clinical trials in order to know how to treat patients most effectively when the drug of choice ceases to be effective. In this regard, the complexity of curing cancer presents a formidable obstacle.

A large number of humans have also undergone mutational profiling to identify gene sequence variations associated with diseases such as obesity, diabetes, Crohn's, and ulcerative colitis, among others. These studies disclose the relative frequency of genetic mutations in afflicted versus healthy individuals. These patterns are extremely valuable to researchers because they illuminate dysfunctional genes, pathways, and/or systems. The findings of these investigations lead to an important conclusion. First, the majority of diseases are complex, and when mutational data is analyzed collectively, the role of numerous genes that, when altered, predispose humans to disease onset and/or progression is revealed. Typically, affected individuals carry mutations in only one or a small subset of these genes, highlighting the fact that defects in a number of distinct pathways are sufficient to predispose individuals to disease. It follows that, although the afflicted share a common disease, only a subset of afflicted individuals shares the molecular explanation for their disease.

This reality is extremely perplexing to scientists in search of cures because it quickly becomes apparent that the paradigm of one disease-one drug or the single molecule approach to treatment, is mostly flawed and that treatment of disease must be tailored to the specific causal relationship between individuals, suggesting that while a single drug may be effective in the treatment of a single patient, multiple drugs may be required to effectively treat that disease across human populations. While this may be disconcerting, our enhanced knowledge of disease risk factors will enable the drug discovery process to adopt novel strategies. In the past, a clinical trial to evaluate a novel drug in which 10% of participants were regarded effective would have been considered a clear failure. In light of current knowledge, we may reevaluate these outcomes as a tremendous triumph. Perhaps 100 percent of afflicted individuals with particular mutations responded favorably to treatment. This is the future of personalized medicine and a cause for increased future optimism.

Not every mutation is created equal

We may recall from our secondary school introduction to genetics and Mendel's peas that traits such as plant height are inherited unequivocally at highly predictable frequencies. This appears to be a departure from how we have previously viewed mutations associated with human disease. This is due to the fact that they are different. It is essential to differentiate between genetic mutations that virtually assure disease development and those that simply predispose an individual to disease risk. Fortunately, mutations that predispose individuals to disease are significantly more prevalent than mutations that assure disease. These risk factors are quantifiable in terms of how much more likely a person carrying a risk factor mutation is to develop a disease in comparison to those without that mutation.

In reality, things are not so straightforward, as risk factors do not always exert their influence independently of other genetic and environmental characteristics. Some mutations may have additive or even synergistic effects, while others may be protective and reduce or eliminate the negative effects of others. The complexity of mutational combinations makes it extremely challenging to identify gene-gene interactions, especially when sequence data is scarce. Sequencing enough human genomes to precisely identify the occurrence and co-occurrence of gene mutations in healthy and diseased human cohorts is one way to disentangle these complexities. This is not a simple undertaking, as it may require the mutational data of as many as one million affected and unaffected individuals. Unfortunately, this number of afflicted individuals is readily available for many of the maladies we will investigate in this book, should they be willing to participate in such studies.

All previous discussion has focused on risk factors in the absence of environmental effects. Before we get there, let's first examine how these risk factors can be conceptualized practically. As we've learned, risk factors are not a definitive indicator of disease onset. Create a future scenario in your mind. You decide to have your genome sequenced, and your physician informs you that you have two mutations that are cardiovascular disease risk factors. Your physician then informs you that these mutations correspond to a 20% increased risk compared to the human population as a whole. After learning this ominous information, you may eventually wonder whether you can do anything about it. In the majority of instances, the answer is unequivocally yes.

Gene-environment interactions.

Focusing on a different form of interaction, which we refer to as gene-environment interactions, is one of the most effective methods to reduce the risk of disease development. For many diseases, this may entail avoiding substances that your body is unable to metabolize. An extreme example is the condition known as hyperoxaluria. These individuals are unable to metabolize oxalate, a compound found in high concentrations in numerous fruits and vegetables, such as spinach. The accumulation of oxalic acid in such individuals is toxic and results in the formation of kidney stones, which may eventually lead to kidney and liver failure and mortality.

Once diagnosed, these individuals must adhere to a diet that is extremely restrictive and devoid of foods that we typically regard as essential for good health. With the assistance of a professional nutritionist, these individuals adopt a modified diet emphasizing healthful foods without oxalate, which enables them to manage their mutation.

Now, let's return to our friend at-risk for cardiovascular disease. Cardiovascular disease is considerably more complicated than hyperoxaluria, with a greater number of genetic and environmental risk factors. Humans who are at risk for developing this cardiovascular disease must also be mindful of their diet and physical activity, as well as avoiding behaviors that promote disease. The scales of probability may tip against you if you continue to consume a high-fat diet, don't exercise, and don't find better methods to deal with tension. Alternately, by consuming a plant-based diet, reducing tension, and engaging in daily exercise, this person may significantly reduce their risk of developing cardiovascular disease.

Reducing the likelihood of developing a disease would necessitate significant lifestyle modifications for the vast majority of individuals. The issue is that virtually none of us possess a genetic crystal ball at present. It is much simpler for all of us to presume that "disease is someone else's problem, I am strong, and I will not become ill." The statistics do not deceive, and we are increasingly deceiving ourselves and jeopardizing our health by holding these opinions. This book makes an effort to present the facts about a variety of significant diseases, with a focus on what you can do about them with your diet and lifestyle. This information is not only for those who wish to maintain their health, but also for those who are afflicted with disease and wish to find complementary approaches to halt or even reverse its progression.

We should all consider ourselves exceedingly privileged to have a second chance for health in the context of many diseases as the errors of the past can be rectified by merely altering our behaviors, habits and routines. The good news is that cardiovascular disease, type 2 diabetes, and obesity, the three diseases responsible for the greatest number of fatalities worldwide, are all reversible.

All chronic diseases covered in this book are caused by a combination of genetic and environmental risk factors. For the majority of individuals, environmental risk factors, such as diet and exercise, that are under their control can render genetic predisposition mostly irrelevant. By altering the behaviors that place you at the greatest risk, you can increase your chances of living a full, active life.

The regular consumption of a plant-based diet favors networks of species that are able to extract the most energy from the available resources.

Chapter 3
The Universe of Bacteria Within: What Benefits Do Microbes Provide?

The preceding chapters provided an overview of what we know about important human diseases that are increasing rapidly in our society. Disease has existed in human civilizations since the beginning of our existence. The loss of life or debilitation due to disease has fueled humankind's curiosity to understand how the human body functions and particularly what goes wrong when we develop disease. Over the last centuries we have amassed a highly sophisticated knowledge of the functions of each of the major tissues and countless details of the molecular complexities operating within the cells of these tissues. Among the major accomplishments made in the past century is a detailed understanding of the molecular basis for many diseases.

Biological systems are not easily predictable.

Despite these monumental advancements, there is still a great deal to learn about how to translate this detailed knowledge into effective treatments. This is not due to a dearth of effort. In contrast to physics and chemistry, biological systems do not operate in accordance with laws that permit the precise prediction of complex phenomena. Biological systems employ a distinct operating system that, while adhering to the laws of physics and chemistry, includes unpredictably variable factors. For every drug discovery endeavor in the world, there exists a group of scientists persuaded that patients could be cured if only we could inhibit the activity of a particular protein. As history has mercilessly demonstrated, this is simply not the case.

Traditional versus Western medicine.

How we "see" disease is one of the fundamental differences between western medicine and systems developed in the East. In Western medical practice, for instance, maladies of the skin or thyroid gland will attract the focus of researchers and clinicians who will investigate in depth what is wrong with your skin or thyroid function. We always find answers to these queries if we search diligently.

The class of drugs used to treat elevated cholesterol exemplifies the practice of treating symptoms rather than the underlying cause of disease. It is well established that elevated cholesterol levels increase the risk of cardiovascular disease-related mortality. Inhibiting a liver enzyme involved in cholesterol biosynthesis, statins reduce cholesterol levels in patients, thereby potentially preserving their lives. Setting aside the potential adverse effects of these medications, they do reduce cholesterol levels. Notably, the drug does not cure the patient, but rather treats the life-threatening symptoms.

The ability to control cholesterol levels is completely dependent on the drug. For some patients, an improved diet is not sufficient to solve the problem and these people have no other choice but to join the ever-growing number of people on the prescription drug treadmill. This conundrum illustrates the short-comings of our perspective of human disease that focuses on symptoms rather than root causes and life-style choices that negate our need for medications.

In traditional systems of medicine, diseases manifesting in the epidermis or thyroid indicate a primary cause in more fundamental systems. Disorders of the kidney may be the cause of cutaneous diseases. To cure the skin condition in this example, one must address the abnormality of the kidney. The saying "all disease begins in the gut" is attributed to the ancient Greek philosopher Hippocrates. Intriguingly, this belief emerged independently in other ancient civilizations that developed sophisticated medical systems, such as Ayurvedic medicine in India and traditional Chinese (TCM) medicine in China. The fundamental principle of these medical systems is to treat the root cause of disease.

Scholars with extensive knowledge of western and eastern medical systems are of the opinion that if you require critical care or surgical treatment, you will be best served in the west, but for chronic diseases plaguing modern society, eastern or traditional practices have much to offer, especially in terms of disease prevention.

A brief history of feces

Given the vast breadth of medical knowledge, it is baffling that a crucial piece of the puzzle was entirely ignored until very recently. It is like living your entire life in a house that you have explored and maintained for decades only to one day discover a hidden door that opens up into a completely new house that you never knew existed. The microbes that live in and on our bodies, referred to as the human microbiome, are indeed what lay on the other side of the door. The excitement and new promise the gut microbiome offers will take time to fully assess, but based on what we know thus far, it may indeed hold the secrets that will instruct us as to how to effectively treat and cure chronic disease.

If the importance of the gut microbiome is true, how is it possible that it was neglected for all of this time? For hundreds and hundreds of years, human excrement has been reviled due to its noxious odor and its association with disease. In the 19th century scientists began to recognize that microscopic bacteria were one of the common causes of infectious disease responsible for countless deaths and epidemics. Some of the most important discoveries in history to reduce disease have related to improved hygiene and practices to deal with human waste.

Romans are credited with devising the first latrines and sanitation systems, as they realized that public exposure to untreated sewage caused disease. Antibiotics, which were discovered in the middle of the 20th century, may be one of the finest medical discoveries of all time, having saved innumerable lives. Given this history and the unambiguous demonstration that bacteria were the causative agents of disease, it is not surprising that we never considered the possibility that the swarming bacteria found in excrement may have therapeutic value. It would seem absurd to consider excrement as anything other than an offensive waste product that should be kept (at the very least) at arm's length from humans.

In the past, there is evidence that this perspective softened somewhat as farmers began using animal manure as fertilizer to enrich the soil and improve crop growth. Even so, it required a courageous scientific mind to conceive of the possibility that the microbes in our intestines and feces might have medical value. Due to their interest in gastrointestinal infectious diseases, microbiologists began to formally research the bacteria found in human excrement. Undoubtedly startling to these pioneers was the conclusion that the vast majority of these bacteria did not possess any potential to cause disease, a conclusion reached after their isolation and detailed study.

A transformative turning point.

As research progressed, it became clearer that healthy individuals harbor an extensive variety of bacteria, the vast majority of which are not pathogenic (capable of causing disease). None of these studies constituted the "eureka" moment of which scientists fantasize, but it became gradually and even imperceptibly apparent that a reappraisal of gut flora was necessary. These pioneers concluded that these bacterial populations are generally innocuous, but it would be some time before anyone considered the possibility that these bacteria might actually be beneficial to human health.

Researchers interested in intestinal microorganisms must have felt like they were counting grains of sand for a couple of decades. The presence of such a large number and level of diversity rendered the decision to investigate one species or another somewhat arbitrary. The advances in DNA sequencing technology were exceptionally well-timed, as the comprehensive characterization of these bacterial communities required technologies that did not exist and were challenging to conceive of even as recently as the 1980s.

Although the study of the human microbiome has no official commencement date or year, it began in vigor at the turn of the 21st century. It is still a relatively new scientific field, but the discoveries made over the past two decades have sparked increased enthusiasm and research efforts. The initial investigations of the human microbiome were, like many other pioneering endeavors, straightforward census exercises designed to answer fundamental questions. In order to avoid confusion and establish fundamentals, the earliest studies of the human microbiome focused solely on samples derived from healthy subjects. This allowed a variety of questions to be answered, as well as the comprehension of the nature of microbiomes.

Questions, questions, questions.

How do microbial communities differ across unique body sites, such as the epidermis, oral cavity, and intestines, was one of the initial inquiries. How do these communities differ within an organism? How similar are the bacterial populations isolated from the same body sites in different individuals? How similar or dissimilar are the microbiomes of people from various countries? How do dietary habits affect the intestinal microbiome? How do microbiomes change throughout a person's lifetime? This list is extensive, and scientists are working quickly to find answers.

Unveiling the mammalian microbiome.

The majority of the human organism is colonized by bacteria. It has been approximated that the number of bacterial cells coexisting with their human host is ten times greater than the total number of cells comprising the human body (1×10^{14} cells). More precise estimates suggest that microorganisms may slightly outnumber human cells, and that whether you are numerically more human or more microbial may depend on the timing of your most recent gastrointestinal movement. In light of this insight, it has been posited that humans may be better understood as meta-organisms that are part human and part microorganism. This strange-sounding perspective contains a kernel of truth, even if this descriptor may simply be a means to generate headlines in the popular press. The evidence that the presence of our microbial counterparts improves our fitness and health as a species continues to accrue. We are not a truly separate organism but a part of a wider community of species.

Microbiota refers to the community of microorganisms inhabiting a particular environment or niche. Bacteria essentially cover the surface of our skin, and they also reside beneath the surface layers of skin, including the sebaceous glands, perspiration glands, and hair follicles. Our tongues, gums, and teeth are also completely covered with bacteria, which, if undisturbed, form dense, multi-cell layer biofilms. If we do not brush our teeth, these can be seen with the unaided eye. Additionally, the vagina is colonized by microorganisms. It is fair to presume that any body site exposed to the environment contains a thriving bacterial community. Even sites long believed to be sterile, such as the uterus, may harbor microorganisms. There are reports that the prostate and breast tissue may also harbor bacterial populations, though this has not been conclusively confirmed.

Best friends forever.

The discovery that microbes present in the oral cavity, gut, skin and vagina were unique provided an early and strong basis that they were the products of intensive natural selection to co-exist with their human host. The fact that microbiomes were not randomly distributed across body sites indicated one of a few possible explanations. First is that microbes colonizing different body sites were being positively selected for by improving host fitness. The second possibility was that our microbiomes were essentially parasitic imposing their existence on its host taking up residence in body sites that provide the most benefit to their own fitness. The third possibility and overwhelmingly prevailing view is that our microbiomes provide benefit their host while simultaneously serving their own needs. This is what is known in ecology as mutualism that depending on its evolutionary success can ensure a harmonious co-existence for millions of years.

The gut microbiome has been declared champion.

Despite the fact that all microbiomes play essential roles in human health and merit sustained research, the bacterial communities of the human gut have received the most attention and are therefore the best characterized. In terms of the number of bacterial cells, the gastrointestinal environment contains by far the most bacteria. From the stomach (10-100 cells/mL) to the duodenum, the first section of the small intestine (100-1,000 cells/mL), the density of microorganisms increases progressively. In the ileum (distal small intestine), the bacterial density dramatically increases to 10 to 100 million cells/mL. Finally, the colon contains the densest bacterial communities. There are 1 x 10$^{11\text{-}12}$ bacterial cells per gram of feces. This represents the highest density of bacteria in any known environment on the planet.

Partitioning of microbial functions along the length of the gastrointestinal tract.

The species found in each segment of the gastrointestinal tract overlap and are also distinct from one another. The distinctive microbiota found throughout the digestive tract are influenced in part by environmental variations in the intestines. For example, an oxygen gradient, where oxygen is abundant in the small intestine, scarce in the ileum, and essentially absent in the colon, favors distinct populations of gut bacteria. Similarly, the pH in the gastrointestinal tract varies along a similar gradient, with the pH being lowest (most acidic) in the ileum and gradually approaching neutral in the distal colon.

Along the length of the gastrointestinal tract, microorganisms act successively on the food we consume. The small intestine absorbs the calories and micronutrients that are most readily extracted from our diet. This transit provides the colonic microbiota with a diet of partially metabolized materials or dietary fibers that the small intestinal microbiota cannot digest. The gut microbiota has evolved to generate a complex set of gut communities that exhibit high levels of metabolic cooperation within their own subcommunities (such as the upper ileum).

Additionally, these site-specific communities collaborate with downstream communities that inhabit the colon. The efficiencies gained by partitioning distinct populations of bacterial species along the length of the gastrointestinal tract may become fixed in a manner that provides stability for all gut communities.

It is estimated that the number of genes encoded in human microbiomes is greater than 150 times that of its host. The extensive repertoire of genes and functions transmitted by the gut microbiome enables humans to be more adaptable, especially in terms of deriving greater benefit from our diet. The human genome, despite being extraordinarily complex, has a fixed composition and, consequently, a limited capacity to adapt to changes in our environment (specifically our diet), whereas the intestinal microbiome has evolved to permit rapid adaptation in response to changing environments.

The gastrointestinal microbiome of an average healthy adult contains 100-200 species of microbes that are readily observable by DNA sequencing. The majority of these microorganisms encode a small number of about 2,000 to 4,000 genes and, as a result, have limited ability to perform functions independently.

Consequently, the viability of microbes coexisting in the human environment is determined not only by the functional capacity of its own genome, but also by the functional capacity of its neighbors.

Cooperation is in high demand for bacteria and this drives the natural selection of larger consortium of species to form complimentary relationships that allow them to achieve greater metabolic potential than any individual species possess on their own. This type of cooperative selection sets the stage for the utopian society that a healthy gut microbiota represents.

More than the sum of its parts.

Depending on the difficulty of the task at hand, the magnitude and complexity of bacterial consortia or interaction networks vary. The bacterial metabolism of simple sugars in the diet does not require cooperation, whereas the metabolism of complex carbohydrates, such as those found in plants, may require the cooperation of multiple species. Let's examine this important form of cooperation in greater detail to better understand how networks form and function.

Dietary fiber consists of complex carbohydrates that are incapable of being metabolized by the host nor imported directly into bacterial cells. Therefore, bacteria-produced enzymes are required to break down these sugar polymers into smaller molecules. A complex dietary carbohydrate may comprise a variety of monosaccharide sugars held together by various chemical bonds. Each unique sugar and chemical linkage must be broken down by a unique enzyme, necessitating the concerted action of multiple enzymes encoded by multiple bacterial species. Therefore, the regular consumption of a plant-based diet favors networks of species that are able to extract the most energy from the available resources. The great diversity of nutrients we ingest in our diets requires that numerous functional networks form within the community to ensure that the energy and nutrient potential of our diet is most efficiently obtained. While the microbes efficiently utilize the liberated sugars for energy, some are absorbed by the host. Indeed, it has been estimated that up to 10% of our daily calories are derived from otherwise indigestible carbohydrates provided by the work of our gut microbiome.

Microbiomes are similar to the communities in which we reside.

The towns and cities in which we reside are populated by people who provide a variety of occupations and services to keep things running efficiently. A greater number of builders, architects, and attorneys, among others, are drawn to thriving cities. A tranquil municipality has little need for a large police force, but it still requires grocery store employees, physicians, and teachers. A large metropolis necessitates more police and firefighters to maintain community safety and harmony. In this manner, the requirements of the villages and cities are ultimately met. Diet is the primary determinant of the tasks performed by microorganisms in microbial communities, which are otherwise quite similar. Dysbiosis, using this analogy, represents a restructuring of the harmonious community as the result of criminals coming to town. This event increases the need for more police and lawyers and so on.

Plant based diets will select for microbes that are distinct from those of a strict carnivore. Each species' abundance in the community varies considerably. One or two species constitute 10-20% of the total community in healthy individuals, where one or two species are typically dominant. The colossal number of bacteria found in the large intestine supports the notion that these species are capable of a vast number of biochemical transformations. These dominant species are complemented by five to ten species with an abundance of 1-5% of the total community. A larger number of 50-100 species display an abundance between 0.01-1% of the total. The abundance of any particular bacterial species is a direct reflection of its overall fitness in that community. Therefore, the secreted products of the most dominant species have the greatest impact on host physiology, whereas less abundant species may only have impact on the host as a collective or consortia of bacteria that may generate the same products.

Brush your teeth after every meal.

Consider how the structure and hierarchy of the bacterial communities in our gut facilitate physiological changes in their hosts. A simple example can be found on our tooth surface where the dental microbiome resides. The profound biochemical capacity of the dominant species present in the human microbiota is exemplified by events which occur mere minutes after our first-morning taste of orange juice. Healthy teeth have a pH of approximately 7.0. The microorganisms on your teeth are experts at digesting sugar.

So vigorous is this activity that the pH on the tooth surface begins to drop within 1 minute of sugar exposure. The rapid metabolism that ensues generates lactic acid that reduces the pH below neutral. Over the course of the ensuing hour, the pH may drop as low as 6.0 but then gradually returns to neutral. The low pH becomes inhibitory to the dental microbiota causing them to slow their metabolism and production of acid.

If we habitually eat too many sweets, we may select for species that are even more proficient at sugar metabolism and resistant to acid inhibition. The change in pH from the same glass of orange juice can become more dramatic and result in a pH on the tooth surface below 5.5, taking longer to return to neutral. At this pH, the acid is strong enough to demineralize the enamel on the tooth surface that over repeated insults may result in tooth decay otherwise known as a cavity and an unpleasant visit to your dentist.

The longer teeth are exposed to pH levels below 5.5, the more demineralization occurs and the more rapidly cavities develop. This is why our mothers insisted we brush our teeth after every meal. Once tooth decay has occurred, the acid-producing bacteria become more dominant, putting other tooth surfaces at risk of a similar fate. This is the reason

Why we are encouraged to visit our dentists twice a year

This example illustrates how our dietary and behavioral practices can alter a healthy microbiota that protects us from colonization by heavy acid producers. Our behaviors have a direct effect on our susceptibility to disease. As with other conditions we will discuss, host genetics factor into the susceptibility equation. Individuals differ in their salivary gland activity and thus the ability to protect the teeth from the effects of acid. Similarly, tooth remineralization is a gradual process determined by genetic factors.

The example in which our resident microbiota contributes to cavity formation and interacts with genetic factors is an example of disease causation by microorganisms that is relatively straightforward. The well-understood process of sugar fermentation by microorganisms resulting in acid production makes it straightforward. The activities of minor species on the tooth surfaces of healthy individuals can shift over time into high-abundance bacteria that drive the onset and progression of disease.

The average of the group.

The more numerous, moderately abundant bacteria present in microbial communities are also of high significance, as they contribute a higher degree of species diversity that confers greater gene/functional diversity on the communities. Gut communities best illustrate the importance of this group of organisms. Diverse dietary compounds are broken down in the stomach as a consequence of the high acidity and acid-tolerant enzymes produced by humans. Proteins are broken down into short amino acid polymers called peptides.

We learned previously that a consortium of microbes is required to degrade complex carbohydrates such as dietary fibers. While glucose is the primary source of energy for most cells in the body, cells lining the colon prefer butyrate, which belongs to the class of compounds known as short chain fatty acids (SCFAs).

This preference may reflect a specific adaptation of these cells to coexist with their microbial counterparts, as numerous bacteria in the large intestine metabolize carbohydrates and produce SCFAs such as butyrate. This is an excellent example of how the host and microbes engage in a mutually beneficial relationship and demonstrates how the activity of microorganisms enables the extraction of additional energy from the diet that would not be possible otherwise.

Calling in the reserves.

A third group of species present in human microbiomes is rarely described because their abundance is so low and they are therefore unlikely to carry out processes that could alter host physiology. Surprisingly, this component of the community is composed of a significant number of species, including 1000 or more diverse bacterial species. Why do these bacteria exist if they have little influence on host or community physiology? The answer to this query could not be deduced from individual samples of microbiota in human feces.

When we investigate the changes in gut microbiota composition before and after dietary change in a time series referred to by scientists as longitudinal analyses, we observe that some species of very low abundance can become part of the more abundant microbiota and vice versa. Imagine a strict carnivore with a gut microbial community selected for efficient utilization of dietary proteins and fats. Microorganisms that are specialized in extracting nutrients from a plant-based diet are present but concealed in populations of extremely low abundance. If our carnivorous acquaintance decides to become a vegetarian, the natural selection would shift favoring microbes specialized in metabolism of a plant-based diet.

These changes perfectly reflect the behavior of microorganisms. Simply stated, they respond to their environment. Some microbes flourish when protein sources are abundant, whereas others thrive on a vegetarian diet. According to studies, changes in the composition of the intestinal microbiota are apparent just one day after a dietary change and continue to evolve into a well-adapted vegetarian community in less than one week.

In this context, the "value" of a species to the gut's metabolism is entirely redefined based on the lifestyle decisions of its host. Imagine if the reservoir of low-abundance species did not exist and the carnivore's intestinal microbiota was permanently optimized for that diet. The decision to become a vegetarian may be detrimental to the host's health, as the resident intestinal microbiota would be ill-equipped to extract energy and nutrients from a vegetarian diet.

Thankfully, the vast diversity of microbes in our intestine, which spans an astonishing abundance range, is highly adaptable, allowing its host to derive the greatest possible benefit from a variety of diets. In this regard, all bacterial species present in our intestine have context-dependent significance. Depending on our dietary and lifestyle choices, a species that is currently of little significance to our health may become crucial to our wellbeing in the coming week. Similar to a well-orchestrated symphony, each instrument and performer has a distinct and vital role to play. Not all of the musicians play at the same time, but when the conductor deems it appropriate, they each contribute their individual talent.

The forces of Darwin's natural selection function swiftly and reliably, enabling us to comprehend why it is imperative that the benefits we derive from our microbial counterparts are determined by what we choose to consume. It may be tempting to believe that our intestinal microbes are robbing us of energy that we could use. If our microbiome received no benefit from our diets, it would be impossible to modify these communities when we alter our diet. It is by virtue of their ability to derive the energy required to multiply that natural selection can drive the changes in microbial composition that best serve our needs. Thus, while the microbes do take their cut from our diet, evolution of humans has included microbiomes since in healthy individuals, they give back at least if not more than what they take.

The vast gene diversity and adaptability of the gut microbiome have allowed us to better appreciate the enormous functional potential of our microbial friends. This appreciation has even led some to compare the gut microbiome to a new human organ. In many ways this comparison is a fair one. The contents of our gut and fecal matter have indeed undergone a dramatic transition in perception from useless, disease-causing waste products to an entity of extreme value and importance in human health. The shared responsibility of metabolism defines a strong signature of mutualism among co-existing organisms.

Fruits and vegetables, the health-promoting foods we consume, are healthful because they contain a variety of molecules with exotic names such as polyphenols, flavonoids, and phytonutrients. We have learned that the biochemical transformation of nutrients by gut microbiota enhances their absorption. As an added benefit, these transformations frequently increase their bioactivity. Bioactivity refers to the capacity of a particular molecule or family of molecules to affect our physiology. Obviously, increased bioactivity of healthy compounds is a positive thing, but increased bioactivity of unhealthy compounds is detrimental to human health and increases the likelihood of developing disease.

While we are beginning to comprehend the specifics of many of the dietary conversions performed by the gut microbiota, the complexity of our diets and the magnitude of the nutrients present make it abundantly apparent that our knowledge of microbial biochemistry is dwarfed by what we do not know. In subsequent chapters, we will investigate in greater depth how our diets alter gut communities and how these alterations can either contribute to enhanced health or, in the case of an unhealthy diet, contribute to disease.

Uniquely you.

Examining the microbiomes of tens of thousands of humans has led to the significant discovery that each individual's microbiome is distinct. It is likely that no two people on the planet have exactly the same microbiome; therefore, our microbiomes are analogous to fingerprints that identify us as individuals and highlight our uniqueness. Unlike true fingerprints, our microbiomes are constantly changing and are therefore not really comparable to fingerprints, but they nonetheless represent highly personalized communities that have evolved alongside us since birth. While intriguing in and of itself, this has significant implications for our health and disease propensity.

Several factors contribute to the uniqueness of our microbiomes. Perhaps surprisingly, our genetics is not a dominant factor of our unique microbiome fingerprint. This was demonstrated by a number of studies that examined the relative similarity of gut microbiota present in identical twins that share an identical genome compared to non-identical twins that only as similar genetically as any two siblings. This comparison demonstrated that the gut microbiota of identical twins was only just slightly more similar than non-identical twins. This result suggests that genetics is not a major contributing factor of microbiome composition.

In light of the fact that twins, whether identical or not, have microbiomes that are more similar than those of unrelated children or siblings born at separate times, these findings are somewhat puzzling. Additional studies have demonstrated that our microbiomes are primarily transmitted through human contact and the surrounding environment. This topic will be discussed in greater depth in chapter 5, but the relative importance of this inheritance may be a determining factor in our lifelong resistance and susceptibility to disease.

Stable as a table.

Stability over time is a characteristic of the intestinal microbiome that came as a bit of a surprise. When gut microbiota communities were surveyed over the course of a year, the profiles remained relatively unchanged. This appears to be a characteristic of fit people who consume a varied, nutritious diet. While the abundance of some species fluctuates at varying intervals over time, these fluctuations tend to be constrained such that their average abundance over any time interval is essentially preserved. Studies investigating this phenomenon over longer periods of time, such as 10 to 20 years, have not yet been conducted, but it appears, in the absence of contradictory findings, that the intestinal microbiota of healthy adults is stable.

The consistency of the intestinal microbiota in healthy individuals provides a valuable comparison framework for other contexts. In what circumstances, for instance, is the microbiome unstable? As we will learn in Chapter 6, the microbiota in the first few years of life is unstable and a reflection of the organism's drive toward a stable configuration. As will be discussed in greater detail in Chapter 8, the intestinal microbiome loses its stability in older individuals. Thus, the microbiota endures alterations relative to that of a healthy adult. In a variety of disease contexts, the gut microbiota endures a variety of alterations, as discussed throughout part 2 of the book.

On the basis of comparisons between microbiota samples obtained from the same body sites, the microbiota of individuals residing in distinct geographical regions of the world are distinct. The American microbiome is distinct from those of Africans and Asians. Dietary cultural differences are likely responsible for the majority of these geographic differences. Asian diets are more likely to include fermented foods, fish, and other foods less commonly consumed in the West. African diets are much less likely to include processed carbohydrates and high-fat foods in large quantities.

Natural selection and bacterial evolution.

Bacterial species are given Latin names that are often times difficult to pronounce and mean very little to the average person, but are based on a system of taxonomy and ancestry that will be helpful to understand a little bit better. Bacteria were the first life forms on the planet, thought to have arisen ~4.1 billion years ago.

For simplicity let's assume that this bacterial cell began to divide passing its genes onto its progeny. This cell division represents an important event from an evolutionary perspective since our world now comprised of two bacterial cells are free to evolve independently. Changes to the DNA sequence of both lineages will occur at random and given enough time, the progeny of the original cells may have uniquely acquired improvements on the genes they hold in common or independently evolved new functions thus achieving meaningful and useful distinctions from their common ancestor.

Eventually enough changes occur to warrant that these progeny define two unique species. This process of cell division and mutation continues over millions of years until two species became four and then eight and so on. Genetic variation is the driving force of biological diversity. The imposing environment existing on early earth applied strong pressure to ensure that these early life forms became efficient and tolerant to environmental insults. Some changes occurring at random jeopardized the cell's existence and were forever wiped out, while other changes benefitted the cell thereby increasing its chances of survival and its ability to pass its genetic material onto its progeny.

We imagine that as life on earth diversified within the microbial world so too did the diversity of functions that allowed some species to adapt to new environments that posed new challenges. The evolution of new functions takes a very long time but as the diversity of functions "invented" by natural selection continued to grow, it became advantageous for bacteria to evolve mechanisms to uptake DNA into the cell from the environment or directly from other cells. These acquired functions may or may not have any value to the recipient cell but this trial-

and-error process patiently conducted over eons of time is the fuel of natural selection and increased fitness.

Share, share, that's fair

Despite the apparent inefficiency of this process, if the acquired function provides a competitive advantage to the recipient, it becomes fixed in the genome and will continue to fine-tune its function by mutation. This process of gene sharing is referred to as horizontal gene transfer and has a dramatic impact on the rate of bacterial evolution since each evolved function need not be re-invented but can instead be temporarily or permanently borrowed from a long lost relative.

Gene sharing is a process that not only speeds up the rate of evolution but also accelerates the trial-and-error process of genome optimization since bacteria occupying the same environment, such as a hot acid lake, have the same evolutionary needs as other species occupying that same environment. Therefore, if a long-lost relative has invented a useful gene conferring resistance to acid or high temperature, it is considerably more efficient to acquire that gene that to re-invent it on your own.

In this regard, evolving mechanisms for sharing and acquiring genes may have been of considerable advantage in early evolution. The ability of bacteria to share and acquire genes from the environment still exists today. This is precisely why antibiotic resistant bacteria are particularly problematic in hospital settings.

Bacteria in hospitals are exposed to antibiotics routinely. The majority of microbes are killed by such exposures but once drug resistant bacteria are present these highly useful gene functions can be shared with other bacteria. By this same process bacteria resistant to a single antibiotic eventually may become multi-drug resistant. So strong is the selective pressure for antibiotic resistance we see just how fast the evolution of drug resistance can evolve in a matter of decades, years and even months. Multi-drug resistant bacteria a.k.a. superbugs have become a major concern of health organizations around the world and yet despite our clear understanding of these processes, antibiotics remain our best existing weapon to safeguard against deadly infectious diseases.

Given the very extended timeframe that bacteria have been evolving, it is perhaps not too surprising that bacterial evolution has generated a fantastic repertoire of species and a mind-boggling number of unique gene functions. It has been estimated that earth is inhabited by 10^7-10^9 unique species of bacteria. These species have evolved an unimaginable diversity of genes that enable microbes to live in some of the most inhospitable environments planet earth has to offer.

Bacteria not only survive but flourish in every environment in which they have been found, including a half-mile deep in the ice of Antarctica, in heated thermal vents with temperatures exceeding 90 °C. Other bacteria have been discovered deep within rocks submerged nearly 1.5 miles beneath the ocean, as well as others in the deepest oceans more than 6 miles beneath the surface. Although these discoveries excite our imagination, they should not be surprising given that bacterial life originated in a hellish ecosystem during the Hadean period.

Selfless microbes.

Evolutionary mechanisms for survival are evident in many forms in bacteria, revealing the selfless nature of microbes. One of the more common mechanisms is induced when bacteria sense a limitation in nutrients in the environment, no longer able to support their growth. Many species of bacteria enter a quiescent or dormant state in such situations, forming spores. Spores are metabolically inactive and highly resistant to environmental insults allowing them to survive for years in this state. Other species take part in a coordinated suicide when the number of cells in the community reaches a high density. Interestingly, this culling affects nearly but not all of the cells in the population, ensuring the survival of the species.

Other species generate slow growth variants in the population ensuring that if the large population of actively growing cells runs out of nutrients and die of starvation, the slow growth variants can survive until better conditions prevail. Most of these mechanisms have been elucidated in pathogenic bacteria that engage in an intricate game of chess with our immune system. While these phenomena may take place in our microbiome, we have not documented such events. However, we do see evidence that microbes in the gut behave in an altruistic manner to sustain their own kind, the community at large and us.

This represents an interesting distinction with regard to the value system of pathogenic microbes that devote a significant number of genes and energy to ensuring the long-term propagation of self, whereas the communities of bacteria in the gut appear to have evolved mechanisms to ensure survival of the community. We will examine some of these mechanisms in the next chapter that illustrate both cooperation within bacterial communities but also how they use their functional potential to help sustain their hosts.

The enormous expansion of gene functions evolved over billions of years have enabled bacteria to adapt to virtually every environmental niche available on the planet and yet only a tiny fraction of these bacteria has the privilege of life in association with humans. Bacteria may well have begun their association with multi-cellular organisms and eventually with animals long before humans existed. An important component of the evolution that took place between the microbes and their host was to form a mutually beneficial co-existence.

A special relationship needed to be struck between these bacteria and the highly proficient immune systems designed to destroy invading bacteria. We will learn much more about this relationship in subsequent chapters as the dysfunction of the harmonious relationship between the gut microbiota and the immune system appears to lie at the heart of a number of diseases plaguing our society today.

It is in the large intestine where microbes are at the highest density that the real biochemical magic takes place, where otherwise useless compounds are biochemically transformed into molecules with increased health benefit.

Chapter 4
The Microbiome: Your Own Personal Nutritionist

Beware and be aware of what you eat.

As a discerning individual, you have developed a commonsense understanding of the foods that constitute a healthy diet and those that do not. However, many of us deceive ourselves into believing that ignoring common sense will not cost us anything. Why is it so? A portion of the reason likely stems from the fact that we do not immediately pay for our lack of common sense. We do not develop disease from a solitary binge of unhealthy foods. Every time we get away with consuming an improper meal, we provide additional evidence that I will be an exception to the rule.

Due to the vast number of systems that maintain homeostasis in our tissues and biochemical pathways, a healthy human body demonstrates remarkable resilience. Negative perturbation, such as a late-night fast-food binge, is managed and absorbed by these systems, enabling the body to maintain healthy functions. Chronic behaviors and poor practices are what subtly throw these protective systems out of sync.

The process of the deterioration of systems safeguarding the maintenance of homeostasis is imperceptible to us, but may begin to manifest in our blood work during our annual health examination. Although the disease has not yet manifested, the writing is on the wall. If you have been told that your cholesterol is too elevated or that you are pre-diabetic and no dietary adjustments are made, you could become a statistic in the future. So, what steps do we need to take to improve our diet and ward off future disease? In order to accomplish this, a crucial first step is to educate ourselves on the types of diet that promote disease and those that promote health restoration.

In pursuit of the perfect diet.

Throughout our lives, we have been exposed to numerous dietary fads and "perfect diet" claims. The ideal diet is coveted and a topic of vibrant, even passionate debate. Paleo, vegetarian, vegan and ketogenic diet advocates appear to have flooded social media with their pronouncements. Concerning these and other diets, both valid arguments and misinformation proliferate. Each diet has advantages and disadvantages. A perfect diet may not exist, rendering those who seek it similar to Ponce de Leon, who is rumored to have unsuccessfully sought the fountain of youth.

Personalization of diets.

Accumulating evidence suggests that the health benefit of different foods and food components may vary widely across individuals. In this regard, nutrition and what constitutes a healthy diet may be highly personalized. Put another way, while a plant-based diet promotes health for all, the overall benefit one person derives from a particular plant may differ significantly compared to another person.

It is becoming increasingly clear that the activities of the gut microbiota are key determinants of which nutrients are most beneficial to our health. Furthermore, gut microbes dictate the magnitude of the health benefit or detriment we experience from our diet. As we have learned, simple dietary compounds and energy are efficiently assimilated in the small intestine. However, the dietary materials entering the colon remain rich in energy content and poorly absorbed nutrient molecules, particularly those present in plants.

93

It is in the large intestine where microbes are at the highest density that the real biochemical magic takes place, where otherwise useless compounds are biochemically transformed into molecules with increased health benefit. We also learned in the preceding chapter that an important characteristic of the gut microbiota is its high variability across individuals. The bacterial species harbored in your gut and whether they belong to the dominant or very low abundance communities are unique to you and define your personal gut microbiota fingerprint. In this sense, your microbial fingerprint dictates the relative health benefit derived from our diets and ultimately defines your personal "perfect diet".

On the basis of these guiding principles, delineating your ideal diet would appear to necessitate a comprehensive accounting of the microbes you harbor and their biochemical skill sets. With this knowledge, a person could theoretically choose foods abundant in nutrients that will be efficiently assimilated and utilized by their gut microbiota. This perspective suggests that an ideal diet is one that flawlessly complements the abilities of your microbiome. Your ideal diet may therefore differ significantly from what your "know-it-all" friend insistently attempts to persuade you of. Is a perfect diet possible at all?

There are two major gaps existing today that prevent us from defining our personal perfect diet. First, most of us don't know our gut microbiota profile and even if we did, the science has not yet advanced sufficiently to allow specific and accurate predictions to be made to the functional capacity of those microbes. Similarly, while we have made substantial strides in our knowledge of the large collections of molecules present in natural foods, we have an imperfect understanding of the health properties of those molecules. The ultimate goal of scientists pursuing this topic is to begin to connect the dots, lots of dots that relate microbial gene function to the biochemical transformation of dietary compounds with the greatest health benefit.

While this may sound like science fiction, all of these limitations can be directly addressed with technology. When technology is the solution to a big problem it is often the case that science fiction becomes reality sooner than we think. A growing number of people have elected to have their personal microbiome profiled by companies who offer this service for a nominal fee. Significant research efforts are underway worldwide to define the functional role of species present in human microbiomes with respect to their capacity to liberate and transform dietary compounds into products that are easily absorbed and achieve high enough concentrations in the bloodstream to have beneficial effects.

Our ability to interpret an individual's gut microbiota profile and translate that into the "perfect diet" recommendation will take time, but all of the pieces are in place to carry out these studies in a purposeful manner. The knowledge we acquire in this regard may be paradigm shifting and usher in a new perspective and opportunity to achieve optimal health through an optimal diet for this and future generations to come. Conceptually, this shift in philosophy emphasizes that we make conscious choices about how to best feed our microbial counterparts that then feed us.

For decades, nutritionists in the food sciences have endeavored to identify and quantify the chemical entities present in the foods we consume. Given the diversity of natural and processed foods consumed by humans, it is understandable that this would be a large undertaking. Still more complicated is determining what happens to dietary compounds after they are consumed. Once it is determined whether the products of metabolism have specific effects on human physiology in terms of health maintenance, disease prevention, and disease reversal, the final piece of the puzzle will be in place.

This is a laborious procedure that bridges numerous scientific specializations. The majority of these efforts have centered on the health-promoting compounds found in a variety of fruits and vegetables, herbs, and medicinal plants that are renowned for their health benefits. The compounds found in superfoods such as kale, goji berries, noni, and pomegranate, as well as regional foods traditionally used by certain cultures to treat disease, have also garnered considerable attention. These studies have begun to validate the health benefits of a variety of ancient medicinal practices' foundational components, including traditional Chinese herbal medicine and Ayurvedic medicine from India.

The majority of these compounds can be placed into a reduced number of classes, which significantly simplifies the situation. This simplification gives consumers a fighting chance of comprehending the knowledge base associated with each category and the most nutrient-dense foods for them. Polyphenols, a large family of compounds found in plants and roots, have been the subject of the most research.

Polyphenolic compounds are present in high quantities in many plants to protect cells from the damaging effects of ultra violet radiation, a natural sunscreen. In humans many of these compounds possess high anti-oxidant potential. Anti-oxidants have proven benefits and protect us from cardiovascular disease, cancer, neurodegenerative diseases and aging among other things.

Researchers in the food sciences have conducted a series of objective studies to characterize these molecules in a wide variety of foods. The studies provide insights about which fruits and vegetables are good sources of these compounds and how various food preparation procedures affect their chemical integrity. Carrots are rich in beta-carotene giving them their traditional orange color. We know that when ingested beta-carotene is converted to vitamin A in the liver. Beta-carotene is also a potent anti-oxidant that helps to protect us from the damaging effects of free radicals and oxidative stress that result from normal metabolism of cells throughout our body. More recently, a poly-acetylene named falcarinol, another potent anti-oxidant found in carrots was identified. Undoubtedly future research will uncover additional and previously unknown virtues of carrots and its nutritional content. These molecules are examples of anti-oxidants that act independently of the gut microbiota to provide a health benefit.

In addition to carrots, blueberries are an excellent source of vitamins and minerals, with a higher vitamin K content than carrots. Anthocyanins, hydroxycinnamic acids (caffeic acid, coumaric acid), flavanols (quercetin), hydroxybenzoic acids (gallic acid), and other phytonutrients such as resveratrol are abundant in blueberries. Some of these compounds may be familiar to you, as an increasing number of anti-oxidants are sold in health food stores today. In addition to their anti-oxidant properties, many of these compounds have additional functions and protective properties.

Some polyphenols have a demonstrated capacity to reduce inflammation, a common hallmark of a wide variety of diseases including, obesity, type 2 diabetes, IBD, IBS, ulcerative colitis, cardiovascular disease and others. Similarly, the study of particular polyphenols plays a role in cardiovascular disease prevention through their ability to improve blood cholesterol. Still other polyphenols have the ability to inhibit the growth of tumors associated with a variety of cancers. You may be asking yourself, "If these compounds have such tremendous health benefits, why aren't they more widely known? Why doesn't my physician include them as part of my health care?"

In the remainder of this chapter, we will investigate some of the reasons why these therapeutic compounds remain relatively obscure, as well as the potential that microbial-based therapeutics have to alter this. In Chapter 3, we learned about the intestinal microbiome and how its composition is subject to natural selection's potent forces. We also learned that, among the factors influencing the composition of gut microbiota, diet was the most influential in determining the communities present in our intestines. In addition, we discovered that the human microbiome has two aspects, one of which, perhaps its most natural, is to contribute to our overall health and well-being, while its other face reflects its ability to promote disease.

The bacterial agenda.

It is essential to recognize that bacteria have no desires or goals. Perhaps it would be more accurate to state that bacteria have only one goal, which is to respond to their environment in an efficient manner to assure their survival. Consequently, bacteria are exquisitely attuned to their environment and have an extraordinary capacity to adjust their metabolic and growth state in response to change. The choice of what we consume is entirely up to us, and bacteria simply adapt to this provision or are outcompeted by microorganisms better adapted to the task. In the most basic sense, this is how diet modulates the intestinal microbiome of an individual.

Lessons from B vitamins.

The study of B vitamin biosynthesis reveals an example of bacterial altruism. Humans rely on B vitamins for health and even survival, but the human genome does not encode genes for B vitamin synthesis. Instead, humans rely solely on exogenous sources, such as diet and the B vitamin biosynthetic capacity of microorganisms, for B vitamins. Importantly, B vitamins are substrates for biochemical pathways that produce essential co-factors such as NAD, FAD, and others that are required by a large number of enzymes with essential functions. Without these cofactors, existence would be impossible.

The extensive DNA sequencing of human microbiomes revealed that numerous gut-dwelling bacterial species lack the genes necessary for the synthesis of at least one B vitamin. This discovery is quite unexpected since all cellular life require B vitamins to function. It is implausible that these species have no need for B vitamins, suggesting a compelling alternative explanation. Either the diet continuously provides enough B vitamin precursors to sustain bacterial growth, or, more interestingly, bacterial species capable of synthesizing B vitamins must actively share them with the incapable. To provide B vitamins to those in need, organisms must synthesize and secrete them into the environment.

The majority of diets contain adequate amounts of B vitamins, making intestinal microbial sources a type of failsafe. However, famine and malnutrition were a reality for prehistoric man and for millions of malnourished and hungry modern people around the world. In the absence of B vitamins from the diet, how did humans or their microbiomes survive? This puzzle prompted researchers to investigate whether bacterial species share B vitamins. These investigations utilized a combination of humanized gnotobiotic mice and *in vitro* fecal microbiota culture procedures. Let's begin by defining what a humanized gnotobiotic mouse is.

Mice may be raised germ free meaning they lack any microbiota. These mice are generated by surgically removing pups from their mothers under sterile conditions where they are then subsequently reared in a sterile environment to maintain their germ-free status. When germ free mice are provided a single microbial species or a complete microbiota, they are said to be gnotobiotic. When the donor fecal material is derived from a human source, the mice are considered humanized.

The gut microbiota of humanized mice contains a mixture of bacterial species including those that encode B vitamin biosynthetic pathways and those that do not. These mice were then provided a diet containing all of the normal nutrients in chow but were devoid of any B vitamin sources. The gut microbiota of these mice remained unaltered by this diet suggesting that the microbes capable of making B vitamins actively share them, allowing those who cannot make their own, to retain viability. The fact that the gut microbiota are essentially unaltered by the B-vitamin deficient diet suggested that the donor species supply B vitamins in sufficient quantities to allow recipient bacteria to maintain their fitness in a competitive environment.

To verify these experimental results, the same fecal samples were cultured in laboratory growth media that lacked single B vitamins or all exogenous sources of B vitamins and the same result was observed. The altruism of B vitamin sharing lends support to the notion that the evolution of human microbiota has been reinforced by mutual dependencies, not just between the gut microbes and their host but also between members of the microbial community. In this regard, human society might take a lesson from our microbial friends who have learned that cooperation and sharing is good for the community benefitting all of its members.

Whether our interest in nutrition is motivated by a desire for improved health or to end world hunger, it seems evident that our creative energies devoted to solving these problems will include the gut microbiome as a central component in the equation of improved health and nutrition. The science of human nutrition is highly complicated and challenging. A simple piece of fruit and its nutrient content is affected by a multitude of factors such as soil quality, geography, genetics, sun exposure, time of harvest and so on.

Which foods are healthy?

There is overwhelming evidence that fruits and vegetables are beneficial to health. This has prompted numerous scientists to pose the logical follow-up question: what molecules in healthy meals are responsible for their nutritional value? A significant objective of nutritional science is to ascertain how these molecules are affected by food processing and high-temperature heating. Furthermore, it is of interest to determine the fate of nutrients once they have been ingested, and determining the nutrient concentrations required to positively influence human physiology may be the most essential and difficult task.

We are beginning to recognize simple measures of the nutrient content of these foods are inconsistent. Moreover, and more importantly, this information is insufficient to accurately foresee how any particular individual will benefit from consumption. Any fruit or vegetable contains tens of thousands of distinct compounds in varying quantities. Research naturally focuses on the molecules that are prevalent in healthful foods. We have identified the compounds that are particularly abundant in certain foods based on decades of research.

Blueberries, for instance, are rich in the polyphenol hydroxycinnamic acid, while plums are rich in coumaric acid and curly kale is an excellent source of quercetin. Quercetin is present in virtually all fruits, vegetables, legumes, tea, and wine, whereas flavanones are derived from citrus fruit, soy, and apples only. Much of this information is restricted to scientific reports that are difficult for non-scientists to comprehend due to the extensive use of scientific jargon. This information is obviously crucial if one wishes to ensure that their diet contains a variety of polyphenols.

The majority of polyphenols are found in the cuticles of fruits and vegetables, despite the fact that they represent a negligible fraction of their mass. In fact, the outer surfaces of fruits and vegetables are inherently exposed to the most sunlight, which explains why these compounds are concentrated in these areas. Manufacturers of processed foods frequently remove the coverings of fruits and vegetables to enhance their appearance, thereby removing the nutrient-dense portion of these foods. In the same way that the hulls of cereals such as wheat contain the majority of the polyphenols that are removed to improve the aesthetic quality of flour, fruit juices are clarified for the same reason, eliminating a significant amount of the nutrients we obtain from their consumption.

We may be deceived into believing that it is acceptable to rely on processed foods and that they are a suitable replacement for fresh, natural whole foods due to the abundance of these foods. In addition, additives and preservatives in processed foods may actually be detrimental to our health. However, we continue to fill our grocery carts with processed food after processed food, sometimes to the exclusion of genuine foods.

Food sciences continue to develop and must now take into account the role of the gut microbiota as a factor that directly influences the actual nutrient content of healthful foods we ingest, as well as the potential harm caused by a typical Western diet. Similarly, to how we can envision a day in the not-too-distant future when the DNA sequence of our genomes will be routinely used to assess our susceptibility to disease, it is likely that individuals will begin to evaluate their own microbiomes. The current utility of this knowledge for both our genome and metagenome is somewhat limited, but over the next decade, our capacity to interpret the vast amounts of DNA sequence data will improve dramatically.

This transition will be accompanied by an increased number of instances of what is known as "actionable" data. Actionable data implies that we not only have the knowledge to interpret the DNA sequence information but also assign prudent therapeutic options to help safeguard your health or reverse diseases. As our understanding of the functional capacity of bacterial species found commonly and uncommonly in human gut microbiota increases, we will similarly be empowered with actionable data that tells us the foods to avoid as well as those that approximate our very own perfect diet. In the next chapter we will further examine the strong relationship between our gut microbes and diet to understand how these unseen collaborators ultimately dictate our health status in the long-term.

Our gut microbiome is our own personal bioreactor, so
when we change our microbiome, we change ourselves.

Chapter 5
Your Diet and Microbiome Have an Inextricable Relationship.

What have we learned about our microbiome?

Despite the fact that our microbial counterparts have unfailingly served us, it has only been within the two to three decades that we have come to truly appreciate this. Let's examine some of the most important aspects of what we've learned about how the gut microbiome influences both the health benefits of a healthy diet and the price we may ultimately pay for consuming an unhealthy diet. In the past twenty years, a flurry of research has significantly advanced our knowledge and perspectives on diet, and, as with any novel science pertinent to a complex phenomenon, this has highlighted how much more there is to learn.

Much of what we have learned about the impact of diet and health and its relationship to gut microbes has been based on experimentation using rodent models. While most animal models fail to provide precise equivalency of human physiology, it appears that what we learn in mice and rats with respect to diet translates quite well and has been very informative in the context of gut microbiota and gut health. While scientific investigations on diet and its health effects are still preferentially conducted in human subjects, there are compelling reasons to opt for animal studies.

Humans are unreliable subjects.

Humans are not the most reliable test subjects. Some dietary studies are administered in such a way that the participant's entire diet during the study period is provided. These studies are generally hampered by a comparatively small number of participants because they are costly to conduct. More commonly, studies involving human subjects are founded on questionnaires that seek to determine your dietary habits by establishing the frequency with which you consume healthy and unhealthy foods. Self-assessment is notoriously flawed, due to inaccurate reporting, most often based on self-deception. People often believe their diets are healthier than they really are. They may over-emphasize in their mind the time they opted for the salad instead of the hamburger, not realizing the actual trends of their eating behavior.

Still other studies permit participants to consume whatever they desire, and then, based on their dietary reports, place them into categories that most accurately reflect their eating behaviors. Another variation is to provide participants with general guidelines regarding how much of certain foods to consume and which foods to avoid during the study period, which are then compared to their diets prior to the study. People have a tendency to forget what they ate on specific days or meals, or they may feel regretful about reporting the foods they consumed that were outside of the guidelines. All of these flaws prevent or impede accurate interpretation of the data and render the study's conclusions generally uncertain.

Despite the desire to research diet in humans, it is frequently impossible to obtain sufficient control over numerous lifestyle variables. Because of this, animal models are utilized more frequently in diet studies. It is much simpler to precisely regulate what and how much rodents consume. Mice in the laboratory do not exhibit genetic heterogeneity, and researchers need not be concerned about the mice's compliance, memory, or honesty.

Mice living in a bubble.

The earliest clues that gut microbes play an important role in how are diets are related to health came from observations of germ-free mice that are reared in a sterile environment and free of any microbial colonization. Germ-free mice have less body fat, greater tolerance of glucose and elevated insulin sensitivity compared to genetically identical, conventionally-raised mice that possess microbiomes.

When germ-free mice are fed a Western diet, characterized by high fat content, high sugar and low or no fiber, they fail to become obese. This key observation strongly suggested that gut microbes somehow play a key role in promoting diet-induced obesity in mice. This conclusion was further supported by studies that colonized germ-free mice with gut microbiota derived from genetically obese mice, diet-induced obese mice and finally obese but not lean human microbiota derived from identical twins, where one twin is obese and the other lean. In all permutations, colonization of germ-free mice with microbiota derived from obese animals or humans conferred obesity to the recipient mice. This is a startling demonstration of the power of the gut microbiota to determine an important physiological trait.

These findings and others motivated numerous efforts to detail differences in the gut microbiota community composition of lean and obese subjects as well as those that assessed the impact of a wide variety of diets and dietary components on gut microbial composition. Taken together, these studies consistently demonstrate the intimate relationship between our diet and our gut microbiome.

Microorganisms respond rapidly to dietary changes.

Since microbes replicate relatively rapidly, dietary changes have the potential to rapidly alter the composition of our gut microbiome. Indeed, this is precisely what we observe. In studies in which human subjects alternate between a plant-based and meat-based diet or a high and low fiber diet for 10 days, the composition of their intestinal community changes in as little as 1 to 2 days. These results demonstrate the significant dynamic influence diet has on gastrointestinal microorganisms and are extremely encouraging for those interested in enhancing their health through dietary changes.

However, the tale is not quite so straightforward. Such dietary interventions demonstrate that not all study participants respond in the same manner. As we already know, every individual possesses a distinct microbiome. The prevalent microbes of a group of lifelong vegetarians have more in common than those of individuals who incline to avoid vegetables. In this example, it is likely that the vegetarian microbiome will respond faster to a particular plant-based diet or dietary fiber than the microbiome of the meat eater. In this regard, an individual's dietary history may ultimately determine how fast the intestinal microbiota responds to dietary changes.

The missing microbes in modern people.

Recent research has revealed a stark contrast in gut microbial diversity between individuals living in developed countries and tribal communities, and diet, in terms of the diversity of plants eaten, plays a key role. Studies investigating the gut microbiomes of people in developed countries have identified a decrease in microbial diversity compared to their counterparts in tribal populations. Factors such as lower numbers of plant species consumed, urbanization, modern sanitation practices, processed food consumption, and antibiotic usage have been implicated in this decline. Reduced microbial diversity is associated with an increased risk of various chronic health conditions, including allergies, autoimmune diseases, obesity, and metabolic disorders.

Studies examining the gut microbiomes of tribal populations living traditional lifestyles have unveiled strikingly high microbial diversity. These communities often have diets rich in plant fibers, whole foods, and a reliance on natural sources. They eat diets featuring a large number of plants and a very wide variety of fruits, vegetables, nuts, pulses, grains, and tubers. Additionally, their exposure to diverse environmental microorganisms, livestock, and close interactions with nature and soil contribute to the acquisition of a more diverse gut microbiome. This heightened microbial diversity may contribute to their reduced susceptibility to certain chronic diseases.

The adoption of Western diets, characterized by smaller varieties of plants, high intake of processed foods, added sugars, unhealthy fats, and low dietary fiber, has been linked to alterations in the gut microbiome. These dietary shifts are often accompanied by a decrease in beneficial bacteria, such as those involved in fiber metabolism. Consequently, the loss of microbial diversity associated with Western dietary patterns may contribute to the rise of chronic diseases observed in developed countries.

Improved sanitation and hygiene practices in developed nations have undoubtedly reduced the prevalence of infectious diseases. However, they may inadvertently contribute to a decline in gut microbial diversity. Excessive cleanliness and limited exposure to diverse microorganisms early in life can hinder the establishment of a robust and diverse gut microbiome. This lack of exposure to microbial stimuli may disrupt immune development and increase susceptibility to certain diseases.

The widespread and sometimes excessive use of antibiotics in developed countries has been a cause for concern. While antibiotics are essential for combating bacterial infections, they can also have unintended consequences on the gut microbiome. Antibiotics disrupt the natural balance of gut microbes, leading to a decrease in diversity and the potential overgrowth of antibiotic-resistant strains. Prolonged or frequent antibiotic usage can have long-lasting effects on gut health.

The differences in gut microbial diversity between developed countries and tribal communities highlight the potential impact of lifestyle, diet, and environmental factors on human health. The reduced microbial diversity observed in developed countries may contribute to the increasing burden of chronic diseases prevalent in these populations. Understanding the interplay between lifestyle choices, microbial diversity, and disease susceptibility can guide interventions aimed at restoring and promoting a diverse and healthy gut microbiome. Acknowledging the significance of gut microbial diversity and its role in human health can guide efforts to promote healthier diets, appropriate antibiotic use, and sustainable hygiene practices to enhance gut health and overall well-being.

Is my poor diet and microbiome reversible?

Many people have consumed diets containing little or no plant-based fibers for long periods of time then switched to a healthier diet for positive gut microbiome impacts. In addition, obese pregnant mothers are known to predispose their offspring to obesity in adulthood. Clearly, the cause of this trait transmission could be complex and involve genetic factors. We also observe that certain microbial genes specialized for the degradation of polysaccharides present in seaweed are significantly more prevalent in human populations that ingest seaweed as a regular part of their diet than in western subjects. So, we may wonder, if my microbiome has been conditioned over the years to cope with a sub-optimal diet, is it reversible? Fortunately, the short answer is yes.

Research has shown that changing from a poor diet to a healthier diet can positively impact the gut microbiome. The gut microbiome is highly adaptable and can respond to changes in dietary patterns relatively quickly, leading to significant improvements in both microbial diversity and species composition. Switching from a poor diet, typically characterized by too few species of plants, high intake of processed foods, added sugars, unhealthy fats, and low dietary fiber, to a healthier diet rich in whole foods, fruits, vegetables, and fiber can increase microbial diversity. As we have learned, a diverse gut microbiome is associated with improved health outcomes and a reduced risk of various diseases.

Dietary changes can also induce shifts in the abundance of specific microbial species within the gut. A healthier diet typically promotes the growth of beneficial bacteria that thrive on dietary fiber, such as *Bifidobacteria, Bacteroides,* and *Lactobacillus.* These bacteria play crucial roles in fermenting fiber and producing beneficial metabolites that support overall gut health.

A poor diet can lead to an imbalance in gut microbial metabolism, favoring the growth of bacteria that promote inflammation and metabolic dysfunction. In contrast, a healthy diet can promote the growth of beneficial bacteria that produce short-chain fatty acids (SCFAs) through the fermentation of dietary fiber. SCFAs help regulate energy metabolism, maintain gut barrier function, and have anti-inflammatory effects.

Additionally, a poor diet can trigger low-grade gut inflammation, which is associated with several chronic diseases. Dietary changes, particularly those emphasizing whole, plant-based foods and a balanced nutrient intake, can help reduce inflammation in the gut. This reduction in inflammation can positively impact the gut microbiome by creating an environment that supports the growth of beneficial bacteria.

Improving the gut microbiome through dietary changes can have broader health benefits. Studies have shown that dietary interventions aimed at improving the gut microbiome, such as increasing fiber intake, have been associated with weight loss, improved insulin sensitivity, reduced risk of cardiovascular diseases, and enhanced overall metabolic health. It is important to note that individual responses to dietary changes may vary due to factors such as genetic predispositions, baseline gut microbiome composition, and overall health status. Additionally, the long-term maintenance of a healthy diet is crucial for sustaining the benefits to the gut microbiome and overall health.

To each to his/her own.

Just as your microbiome is your own and unlike anyone else's, so too is the responsiveness of your gut microbiome to dietary change. This is most clearly evident in dietary intervention studies that examine a single dietary component, such as the addition of a single plant starch to the diet. This type of study reveals and emphasizes the high variability in the response of the gut microbiota among individuals. These results may have been surprising when first observed, but when we consider how unique our microbiomes are it makes a great deal of sense that the responsiveness to a particular macronutrient would vary.

Scientists tend to track the behavior of bacterial species with their Latin names and potentially draw false conclusions pertaining to the differences in which bacteria were positively and negatively impacted by a particular intervention. In reality, many disparate and unrelated bacterial species may share specific functional capacities; therefore, the apparent disagreement between two compared microbiota on the species level may in fact be the same, if only we understood in better detail the functional capabilities of the two seemingly different species.

If the proportion of microorganisms capable of utilizing a particular polysaccharide is relatively low, let's say 10% in human populations, it is expected that only a subset of microbiomes will respond. Consider a hypothetical experiment in which 10 distinct polysaccharides are administered to the same group of subjects. Also, let's presume that the proportion of microorganisms capable of utilizing each polysaccharide is 10%. This intervention is anticipated to produce a very distinct outcome, with virtually all participants in the study exhibiting a change in their microbiome and virtually no one failing to respond.

The investigators of human health.

Let's examine another well-studied example illustrating how our diet is personalized. The critical work of epidemiologists who study health and disease trends has significantly advanced our understanding of health and disease. The objective of epidemiologists is to understand population differences that correlate with, for instance, the incidence of cancer. This is not a straightforward process and requires an enormous amount of information.

In their pursuit of meaningful relationships, epidemiologists must examine every possible avenue. Differences in genetics and gene mutations are a common starting point; the quality of the air and water must be accounted for; dietary habits must be documented; and even subjective information regarding a person's level of happiness or connection to friends, community, and religion is relevant and considered.

It is essential to recognize that the relationships epidemiologists pursue are rarely of a singular nature, especially in the case of complex human diseases such as cancer. While some of these relationships may ultimately prove elusive, others are so robust that they become distinct hypotheses requiring additional testing and validation. Such was the situation with soy and its potential protective effects against breast cancer in women.

The soybean hypothesis.

To determine why the incidence of breast cancer in Japanese women is considerably lower than in the United States and other countries, an intensive epidemiological investigation was conducted. Although breast cancer incidence frequently has a significant genetic component, this did not appear to explain the difference in breast cancer incidence between the two countries, as Japanese women who emigrate from Japan acquire the breast cancer risk of their adopted country. This is frequently the case with maladies that have a substantial environmental component.

This data led to the hypothesis that the higher soy consumption of Japanese women, may account for the reduced breast cancer incidence in Japanese women. Not only do Asians consume more soy than Americans on a daily basis, but the majority of soy in the American diet comes from processed soy used as filler in a variety of foods. This hypothesis was plausible given that soy contains large levels of phytoestrogens, which are steroid hormones. Chemically comparable to human estrogen, these molecules can bind to and activate the human estrogen receptor. These indicators suggested that the estrogenic compounds in soy inhibit the development of breast cancer.

Therefore, the association between soy consumption and breast cancer appeared far too plausible to be false. As a consequence, a flurry of research aimed to directly test this hypothesis and enhance our understanding of the compounds present in soy, how they are metabolized, and their effect on estrogen-regulated pathways known to be involved in breast cancer moved forward. Unfortunately, discoveries of this magnitude and significance are frequently reported in the popular press before they have undergone sufficient scientific testing to confirm their accuracy. Consequently, goods such as tofu entered our consciousness and vocabulary. Individuals concerned with their health began to incorporate these ingredients into their diet.

Not all microbiomes like soy.

Ultimately these investigations turned to questions pertaining to the gut microbiota that proved to be of high interest in their own right. Two compounds present in soy in high concentration are known as genistein and daidzein. These molecules are chemically similar and their metabolism was studied intensively. Experiments revealed that neither of these compounds were well absorbed in either the small or large intestine, nor were either particularly potent modulators of human physiology. While this may be surprising, it is not at all uncommon.

For instance, it was determined that daidzein is metabolized into two compounds known as O-DMA and equol, both of which are more readily absorbed and

125

possess substantially greater bioactivity. The production of O-DMA and equol is dependent on the activities of the gastrointestinal microbiota present in the colon. This is a second important discovery that has become widely accepted. Third, and perhaps most significant, was the realization that only a small portion of the human population harbors the microorganisms responsible for these biochemical transformations.

About 80% of subjects in the United States have the ability to produce O-DMA, while only 30% can produce equol. Intriguingly, these values are higher in Asian subjects. In addition, the concentrations of O-DMA and equol produced by humans are highly variable and frequently insufficient to have a significant physiological effect.

While research on the potential protective effects of soy, equol, and O-DMA continues, existing evidence does not conclusively support the seemingly logical hypothesis that soy reduces the risk of developing breast cancer. While the excitement surrounding soy has thus far failed to account for any anti-cancer properties, the extensive research surrounding this topic has yielded unexpected but critically important insights regarding the gut microbiota as the ultimate determinant of which foods and dietary supplements are beneficial to your health and which are a waste of money.

In one investigation, the effects of soy processing on a mouse model of breast cancer were investigated. Soy flour, crude soy extracts, and mixtures of purified compounds were fed to mice. The least processed soy flour neither stimulated nor inhibited breast tumor growth, whereas the other forms of soy stimulated tumor growth. Significantly, the processing level of impure extract versus purified compounds was correlated with tumor growth. There are numerous methods to interpret these findings, but they suggest that plants that promote health may do so due to their molecular composition. By manipulating the relative proportions of dietary components during food processing, we may inadvertently destroy or diminish their health benefits. At this time, we do not know the precise answer to this important question, but a number of ongoing efforts are being made to isolate the therapeutic benefits of fruits and vegetables. The question remains, does the purification of single components of healthful foods provide the expected health benefits of the food item from which it was derived?

The miracle compound.

Increasing efforts are being made to convert the molecules found in fruits and vegetables into drug-like molecules. It remains to be seen whether these studies will be viewed as a significant turning point in the revolution of natural therapeutics or as an exercise in futility. In an effort to identify the super molecule capable of curing human disease, researchers are conducting a growing number of studies with this objective. Early findings have highlighted the variable nature of the human gut microbiome in this equation, as many refined molecules are indeed transformed by the gut microbiota to increase their absorption and/or their ability to modify human physiology. However, these transformations are observed in some individuals but not others the majority of the time.

It is essential to differentiate between solitary dietary molecules and complex, fruit- and vegetable-rich diets. While it is possible that some molecules in whole foods are present or assimilated in concentrations that are insufficient to produce a therapeutic effect when consuming standard dietary portions, this is not the case for all molecules. On the surface, the reasoning behind identifying the most therapeutic molecules and concentrating them is sound, but caution must be exercised and additional scientific research must be conducted.

In the meantime, it is evident that adopting a healthy diet that includes a variety of fruits and vegetables will present your gut microbes with thousands of macronutrients, some of which will be ignored while others will be gratefully consumed by bacteria that produce health-promoting substances. These dietary practices enable "good" microbes to outcompete "bad" microorganisms that contribute to obesity and other chronic diseases over time. There is no way to lose by choosing to consume a nutritious diet. There is no way to be completely unresponsive to a healthier dietary change.

In conclusion, the miracle pill may be nothing more than a fiction, whereas there is abundant evidence that a plant-based diet consisting of a wide variety of plants can improve your health and even rectify diseases such as obesity and type 2 diabetes. There are those that believe that distilling a fruit or vegetable down to single molecules is pure folly and instead believe that mother nature has provided fruits and vegetables with a proper balance of healthful compounds, indeed many tens or hundreds of compounds. In this thinking, these compounds are most healthful when consumed together in the original proportions and synergies provided by the food. In other words, health is best obtained and maintained the old-fashioned way, not by eating a pill.

Teach your microbes to eat their vegetables.

One of the most thoroughly researched advantages of adopting a plant-based diet is our knowledge of how gut microbes convert dietary fiber into products that improve human health. We've discovered that the fermentation of dietary fibers is a highly collaborative process involving numerous bacterial species. First, bacteria must degrade the complex polysaccharides (fiber) into simpler oligo, di, and monosaccharides, which can then be selectively transported into bacterial cells to produce energy.

The byproducts of this fermentation are short chain fatty acids (SCFAs), which include butyrate, propionate, and acetate. The proportions of these SCFAs depend on the fibers being metabolized and the number and type of microorganisms in the intestines that are responsible for fermentation. The basic carbohydrates that are metabolized produce SCFAs, which are then secreted as metabolic end products. As the saying goes, "one man's trash is another man's treasure," as these SCFAs are sustenance for other microorganisms that are "bottom feeders," but more importantly, they are essential metabolites for their host. We will learn more about the beneficial properties of these metabolites in the sections that follow.

Examining the microbiota of human populations whose diets are abundant in complex polysaccharides reveals a greater proportion of genes in their microbiomes with the ability to metabolize dietary fiber. In comparison to human populations ingesting a Western diet deficient in dietary fiber, these populations produce a higher level of SCFAs. A multigenerational study in mice fed a Western diet high in fat and low in fiber revealed gastrointestinal microbiota with decreased diversity and proportion of genes coding for polysaccharide degradation.

There is still much to learn about the effects of SCFAs on human health, but the majority of what we do know suggests that these microbial byproducts are crucial for maintaining gastrointestinal health. Butyrate is the primary source of energy for the cells lining the colon; depriving these cells of the energy they need to perform their vitally important function of maintaining a correct barrier between the gastrointestinal contents and the gut immune system has detrimental health effects. Consistent with this, it has been demonstrated that SCFAs improve gut barrier function in "leaky gut" animals and humans. In Chapter 8, we will learn more about the condition of leaky gut and its health consequences.

Butyrate has been shown to alter host gene expression and is able to induce the maturation of immune cells that promote anti-inflammatory responses. Inflammation is a common property of virtually all of the diseases we will discuss in Part 2. This is most likely at least a partial explanation of the protective effects butyrate has with respect to colon cancer development. Propionate and acetate act more so outside of the gut and influence cellular energetics in the liver and other tissues that impact pathways involved in energy expenditure, fat production and fat metabolism. We will revisit this topic in greater detail in Chapter 9.

What microorganisms provide, they can also take away.

The preceding paragraphs highlight the ways the gut microbiota transform components of a healthy diet into molecules that positively influence health. However, as we have alluded to, provided an unhealthy diet, microbes are also capable to increasing our risk of disease through their metabolic activities. One of the best examples of this is based on the less-than-predictable influence gut microbes have on cardiovascular disease risk. One might reasonably ask how do bacteria in the gut influence, cardiovascular health?

The future of microbiological diagnostics could arrive sooner than expected. We now know that gut microbes may metabolize diets high in carnitine (common in red meat) and phosphatidylcholine (common in meat and cheese). Similar to previous examples, the specific microorganisms capable of carnitine and phosphatidylcholine metabolism are not pervasive but are present in a portion of the human population. We do not yet have a complete understanding of the microbes and gene functions that are capable of metabolizing carnitine and phosphatidylcholine, but they are the subject of intensive research as their identification may serve as an effective diagnostic to alert those who should avoid consuming a diet rich in these dietary components.

Trimethyl amine, or TMA, is produced through the microbial metabolism of these dietary compounds such as L-carnitine, choline, and phosphatidylcholine. Once produced, TMA is transported to the liver, where enzymes metabolize it into trimethyl amine oxide (TMAO). Blood TMAO levels are the most accurate predictor of cardiovascular health. There is a direct correlation between elevated TMAO levels and accelerated atherosclerosis (plaque accumulation in the arteries) and the likelihood of severe cardiovascular disease such as heart failure. Vegans who consume no animal products produce minimal levels of TMA.

Rethinking what we thought we knew.

Given our very recent understanding of the relationship between variation in intestinal microbiota and diet, we are in a position to reconsider a number of previously reached conclusions. Consider the number of pharmaceutical medications that performed exceptionally well in animal studies but failed in human clinical trials due to inconsistency in efficacy. How frequently can these failures be explained by the variable presence of gastrointestinal microorganisms encoding proteins capable of altering the drugs, thereby rendering them ineffective in a large proportion of subjects, but highly effective in other individuals?

The evolution of our understanding of such topics has led us to recognize that the response of human populations to diet and medication is not always uniform. It is possible that effective medications to treat human disease have been discovered but have been abandoned due to the high variability of treatment outcomes. This possibility suggests that "failed" medications should be reevaluated in the context of an individual's intestinal microbiome to determine which are most likely to be effective. This is precisely the mentality of modern pharmaceutical companies, which recognize that not all colon malignancies, for instance, respond well to a particular treatment.

Personalized medicine is the biomedical frontier of the future and the future of medicine. Perhaps it is only a question of time before pharmaceutical companies consider gut organisms as a relevant factor in treatment outcomes. There are more reasons than ever to improve our ability to interpret the specific constituents of the human gastrointestinal microbiota, not only in terms of "who is there" but also their biochemical potential.

Given the strong relationship between gut microbes, our diet and a robust immune system, it follows that our dietary choices that maintain healthy microbial communities ultimately impact our immune system health.

Chapter 6
Your Microbiome and a Robust Immune System

We have learned that human evolution has taken place from its origins in concert with microbial populations that colonize our bodies. We have also learned that one of the major driving forces of this co-existence is the added benefit we derive from our diet, based on the immense biochemical transformation capacity encoded by our gut microbiome. A second critical driving force of this co-evolution is reflected by the benefits our immune systems derive through its unceasing communication with gut microbes. Similar to the relationship between gut microbes and our diet, the relationship between the immune system and the gut microbiota is also a story of duality.

The relationship between the intestinal microbiota and immune system is harmonious and beautiful when functioning correctly. When it is broken, it is far from harmonious and resembles a full-scale war in many ways, including assaults, counterattacks, defensive postures, collateral damage, etc. As in any conflict, there are no victorious parties, only losers. This war may last for years at the expense of the health of the populace. In this chapter, we will gain a better understanding of how the immune system functions in health and why it can create havoc in the context of disease states by learning the fundamentals.

The diet-microbiome-immune system axis.

Our immune system is marvelously complex and a description of it is well beyond the scope of this book, however given the number of prevalent chronic human diseases involving immune dysfunction, it is worthwhile to understand some basic principles pertaining to how our immune systems behave in the context of both health and disease. Given the strong relationship between gut microbes our diet and a robust immune system, it follows that our dietary choices that maintain healthy microbial communities ultimately impact our immune system health. In this chapter, we will explore these connections in greater detail.

For most people, the immune system is an enigmatic entity that is only vaguely understood as a defense against infection. We may also be aware that this protection involves the immune system's ability to produce antibodies that eliminate foreign invaders from our bodies. Indeed, these perceptions are accurate, but they do not adequately account for the functions or dysfunctions of the immune system that are responsible for the unprecedented prevalence of chronic disease in modern societies.

The immune system can be divided into two main arms called adaptive immunity and innate immunity. Additionally, the adaptive immune system can be subdivided into two parts: humoral immunity, the more familiar type that generates antibodies to antigens, and cellular adaptive immunity such as in the case of T cells. We will learn more about the latter, as its importance to intestinal microbiota and chronic disease is the greatest.

The immune system identifies pathogenic bacteria and viruses as foreign invaders when they pose a threat to the body. This realization initiates a cascade or chain of events that serve to halt the progression of the infection and purge our bodies of the unwanted guests. It is a true contest between two opposing forces; if the infectious agent prevails, we may succumb to the infection. Fortunately, and as we have all witnessed in our lifetimes, the immune system typically prevails and restores us to health and our regular daily routine. An interesting question that arises that remains a subject of active scientific exploration, is how does the immune system recognize something that is foreign?

The answer to this query is quite complex, but a simple response will suffice for our purposes. In a healthy state, the immune system has evolved to be familiar with all of the proteins, lipids, and carbohydrates in the body. This discovering of "yourself" occurs during fetal development. The immune system recognizes these macromolecules as "self" through a poorly understood mechanism, allowing it to establish what is known as immune tolerance.

In the absence of tolerance, the immune system would not be able to distinguish self from non-self and would launch an unrelenting attack against our healthy bodies. In autoimmune diseases, even a partial collapse of tolerance has devastating, life-altering, and sometimes fatal consequences.

Since our immune system is self-aware, it is somewhat simpler to comprehend how foreign entities are identified. Components of the invader known as antigens induce the production of specific antibodies that bind to the foreign antigen (typically a protein) to neutralize the pathogen and designate it for destruction by other immune cells of the innate immune system that are specialized for this task.

Once the adaptive immune system has been exposed to a specific invader, such as the measles virus, it establishes a long-term memory so that, upon a second encounter, it can quickly and effectively protect us against the insult. This is the premise of vaccination, which is designed to expose us to harmless variants of lethal pathogens in order to protect us if we ever encounter the real thing.

When the adaptive immune system is functioning appropriately, its remarkable efficiency and precision are rarely noticed. In the case of certain allergies, the adaptive immune system can malfunction by mistaking innocuous antigens for lethal invaders. In a similar manner, the adaptive immune system may become maladaptive and mount responses to self-antigens, which are expressed by human cells. The recognition and immune response to self-antigens is known as autoimmunity.

As we have learned, the prevalence of both allergy and autoimmunity in our society has increased dramatically in recent years, prompting a flurry of research efforts aimed at determining the cause of this increase and potential countermeasures. In the next chapter, we will discuss this phenomenon in greater depth in the context of the hygiene hypothesis, which suggests that changes and extinction of species in our intestinal microbiota may increase our susceptibility to these diseases.

The innate immune system also plays an important role in protecting us from infections, but, unlike the adaptive immune system, it lacks memory and can respond to intrusions with a less specific response. The innate immune system takes a more straightforward approach, recognizing that something is "wrong" and unleashing its fury to remedy the systemic breach. In this respect, the innate immune system is analogous to a thermostat that does not care why a room is heated up; it simply responds by cutting off the heat or increasing the air conditioning.

Immune homeostasis: peace and tranquility.

The innate immune system has a more intimate relationship with our gut microbiota, and the study of this relationship has yielded a number of crucial insights into how gut microbes support a healthy immune system. This state of equilibrium is known as immune homeostasis. In contrast, an imbalanced intestinal microbiota can disrupt the innate immune system and contribute to the development of disease. This discordant relationship has been documented in a large number of chronic diseases that will be discussed in the second section of this book. Additionally, it is now evident that when the immune system is compromised, it has the ability to modify the intestinal microbiota. Frequently, this modification results in a dysbiotic microbiota that exacerbates the immune disturbance.

To fully understand how high-density microbial populations are able to coexist with our immune systems, which are specifically designed to protect against bacterial infections, it is helpful to acquire a better understanding of the intestinal environment's architecture. Our gastrointestinal tract is remarkably lined with a single layer of epithelial cells that cover the gut immune system. The epithelium is not a simple, flat, two-dimensional structure, but rather consists of villi, which are rounded peaks and valleys. When observed from above, the villi resemble brush bristles.

This cellular architecture generates a very large surface area, estimated to be between 150 and 300 square meters previously. Recent revisions to this estimate indicate that the surface area of the gastrointestinal tract is between 30 and 40 square meters. Previous estimates were based on cadavers, in which the epithelium appears to lose some of its turgidity, thereby increasing its apparent surface area. The use of modern technologies on living subjects yielded estimates that were considerably reduced but still enormous. The adaptation of gastrointestinal tracts with an increased surface area permits maximal absorption of extracted calories and micronutrients.

A vast array of immune cells and immune cell compartments lie beneath the protective epithelial cell layer. It has been estimated that 60-70 percent of the immune cells in the human body are devoted to the environment of the gastrointestinal tract, highlighting the critical significance of protecting this vital organ system. After all, we cannot subsist if we cannot digest our sustenance.

We can assume that a primary reason for devoting so much immune function to the gut environment is its proximity to an astounding number of bacterial cells exceeding 1×10^{11} per gram of colon contents. This proximity cannot be taken casually, as a breach in the epithelial barrier would enable normally innocuous gut bacteria to enter these immune compartments. Such contact would result in a dramatic immune cell overstimulation and acute inflammation. Immune compartments are vascularized; therefore, the presence of bacteria would overwhelm defense systems and provide a route for bacteria and all of their antigens to become systemically dispersed throughout the body, resulting in a relatively rapid death.

Practice makes perfect.

There are two significant ramifications of the situation described in the preceding paragraph. First, the human immune system has coexisted with intestinal microorganisms and our ancestors for as long as humans have existed and long before that. These eons of time have permitted extensive fine-tuning, which has likely led to the exclusion of bacterial species that were too aggressive and perturbed the immune system in favor of species that the immune system found less objectionable. Over extended periods of evolution, the human gut co-selected for species that were equipped to benefit and flourish in the feast or famine gut environment with which early man had to contend.

The second important implication of the proximity of the gut microbiota and the gastrointestinal immune system requires some understanding of ecological principles pertaining to mutualism. Co-existence is a give and take proposition. Given the massive quantities of energy expended to maintain immune function, it may be safely assumed that the gut microbiota must be providing something of sufficient value to justify the relationship. Over time, the gut microbiota evolved to co-exist with the host. This was most efficiently accomplished by adopting a cooperative assemblage of microbes that establish webs of cooperation that lock into place the feature of community stability that may best serve their host.

By investigating further, the structural characteristics that define the interface between bacterial populations and immune cell compartments, the true nature of the interaction between the gut microbiota and the immune system is revealed. Multiple mechanisms have evolved within the immune system to ensure that interactions between the two occur at a distance. Direct physical contact of cells is undesirable. Mucin, a gelatinous substance that coats the gut lining and is secreted in large quantities by specialized cells lining the intestine, serves

145

to protect the gut lining. This protective layer acts as a physical barrier between microbes and host cells. This polymer covering has two distinct layers, an inner mucin layer with a high density and an outer layer with a low density.

Mucin is composed of a protein that becomes extensively decorated with complex carbohydrates that give mucin its gelatinous character. Interestingly, the composition of sugars present in the mucin layer positively select for specific subsets of the gut microbiota that are capable of feeding on the outer, low-density layer. The inner dense layer acts as a reliable barrier to prevent further bacterial penetration. The structure of this layer presents an interesting dichotomy. The outer layer provides a valuable service in the form of high energy-content food for bacteria, while the inner, dense-layer functions to specifically to limit how close bacteria are allowed to get to the host gut epithelium lining.

While it has yet to be proven to be the case, it is likely that the population of bacteria that forage on the mucin layer are enriched for bacterial species that engage in active communication with the immune system. As these bacteria feed on the outer mucus layer, they become embedded in it. In this regard, their existence may become immobilized in contrast to the luminal populations that go with the flow through our digestive tract until they are ultimately sacrificed to the porcelain plumbing.

Paneth cells, a specialized cell type of the epithelium that secretes a variety of anti-microbial peptides that, like antibiotics, inhibit the development of bacteria in a concentration-dependent manner, are used by the immune system to ensure a relationship at a distance. The structure of the mucin layer contributes to the formation of an antimicrobial peptide concentration gradient. The highest concentration of anti-microbial peptides produced by Paneth cells is found at the interface of the epithelium and inner mucin layer, with concentrations decreasing in the outer mucin layer and gastrointestinal lumen. Similarly, Goblet cells in the epithelium produce and secrete significant amounts of antibodies into the mucin layer, creating a similar concentration gradient. These antibodies bind to bacterial surfaces and even encapsulate them. Antibodies may prevent bacteria from penetrating the mucin barrier and gaining access to the epithelium and underlying immune compartments by coating bacteria.

The relationship between the intestinal microbiota and the immune system represents an enormous evolutionary triumph. An innovative solution has been developed that allows us to take advantage of the enormous functional potential of gut microbes while minimizing the risk associated with an intimate relationship. A comprehensive understanding of this relationship highlights the immense benefit that microorganisms provide to our immune system. There is still much we do not comprehend about these relationships, but accumulating evidence demonstrates how changes in intestinal microbiota composition alter immune function.

On the basis of numerous investigations, it is now certain that the communication between the intestinal microbiota and the immune system is two-way. In general, the immune system regulates and maintains the equilibrium of microorganisms in the community. Newborns' immune development and maturation are stimulated by a vast array of signals produced by the intestinal microbiota. In addition, gut microorganisms enhance the immune system's ability to maintain a constant "awareness" of the relative level of risk in the local environment. Importantly, microbial-generated signals can activate or inhibit specific cellular components of the immune system, thereby pushing the immune system towards either pathogenic inflammatory or therapeutic anti-inflammatory responses.

These observations underscore the enthusiasm surrounding the therapeutic potential of microbiome-based and microbiome-produced "drugs". As our understanding of the specific bacterial species capable of stimulating various immune responses improves, we may be able to prevent and reverse a variety of inflammatory diseases and cancers by utilizing natural microbial-based drug strategies.

The plot thickens.

Extensive research has elucidated a complex set of sensing mechanisms operating in intestinal epithelial and immune cells. Several types of host cell surface receptors and cytoplasmic receptors bind to particular bacterial or virally produced products. Continuous sensing of the microbiota provides the immune system with crucial feedback. Mutations in the sensing machinery are prevalent and predispose individuals to IBD and other inflammatory diseases to develop disease.

Establishment of immune equilibrium.

The immune system has evolved a number of complex interconnected systems to maintain immune homeostasis. This system has more checks and balances and redundancies than NASA, all of which are designed to maintain immune homeostasis by balancing its protective capacity and destructive potential. The gut microbiota contributes significantly to this physiological equilibrium. Perhaps somewhat surprisingly, the immune system is not turned off at stable state or what we could call "rest."

The gut epithelium and gut immune system continuously assess the antigens in their environment as part of the immune system's ongoing surveillance efforts. In a nutshell, immune cells perceive these antigens in a binary fashion. Either the antigen is perceived as familiar and non-threatening, or as foreign and potentially dangerous. Continuous sensing of microbial molecules in the gut subtly activates the immune system, resulting in a state known as benign inflammatory tone. In this condition, the immune system is neither dormant nor actively attacking. By maintaining a state of low-level activation, the immune system is primed to launch an aggressive attack in response to a threat. A healthy, well-balanced intestinal microbiota produces a specific number and type of antigens that help maintain inflammatory tone and signal to the immune system that all is well. However, when changes in the composition of the intestinal microbiota occur, the amount and type of antigens produced may also change. These alterations are acutely perceived by the intestinal immune system.

This understanding has been essential in elucidating how the regular ingestion of a western diet not only alters our gut microbiome, but also has the potential to modify the steady-state activity of the immune system. To comprehend the significance of this, it is instructive to consider the effects of inflammation on our tissues, not only those residing in the gastrointestinal tract but those throughout the entire body.

When pathogenic microorganisms invade the intestine, the immune system launches a full-scale assault. Immune cells at the site of an infection produce cytokines, which cause inflammation, and chemokines, which recruit additional immune cells from far away. This inflammatory response is so aggressive that collateral injury is incurred. The recruited immune cells are specialized cells capable of a variety of functions, such as engulfing and destroying the invading bacteria or virus, bolstering the inflammatory response, and actively participating in clean-up efforts.

The orchestration of events is one of the many miracles of the human body and is beyond astonishing. The immune attack is relentlessly aggressive until the battle is overcome. The rate at which the immune system can launch an attack during an infection is of utmost importance, as in many instances it is a race against time to contain the rapidly proliferating and advancing infectious agent before it overwhelms us. Thankfully, the immune system typically wins this contest. Due to the harmful effects of the immune response, it is equally essential that the immune system can shut down quickly once the threat has passed. Why is it so?

In order to purge the body of foreign threats, inflammation is necessary; however, the immune system's activation results in collateral tissue injury due to activated cytotoxic cells and factors that induce cell death. Once the infection is under control, the body engages in active tissue repair processes during acute inflammation, with minimal or no long-term consequences. Chronic low-grade inflammation, despite being less detrimental, is frequently systemic, as in the case of obesity, making it potentially more difficult to recruit immune functions involved in tissue repair because minor battles are occurring in multiple locations.

All of the diseases to be discussed in the second section of the book involve chronic inflammation, which, even at low levels, poses a serious threat to our health and, over time, can cause irreversible tissue damage and alter the physiological function of various tissues and organs, thereby promoting disease development. Inflammation is the adversary, and while an imbalanced microbiota in the gut, such as pathogens, can induce inflammation, a healthy microbiota can dampen these signals by triggering anti-inflammatory processes.

Gut dysbiosis.

The composition of the intestinal microbiota is considered dysbiotic when it differs significantly from that of healthy individuals. This appears to be a rather imprecise definition, and indeed, it is. Given what we know about the natural variation of gut microbiota between individuals, it should not come as a surprise that distinguishing dysbiosis from natural variation is difficult and problematic. Some gut dysbioses are obvious and straightforward to identify, whereas others are more subtle.

To illustrate how gut dysbiosis is defined we may consider the following example. If the gut microbiota of 100 healthy individuals is sequenced or "profiled", we may learn that the abundance of *E. coli* is between 0.01-0.1% in most subjects and is never observed to be above 0.5% of the total microbial population. With this information we have a framework to establish a normal range and therefore also what we may view as abnormal. If the same holds true for 1,000 and then 10,000 healthy subjects, the framework strengthens and the more certain we can be that a person with *E. coli* abundance of 6% is abnormal and worthy of being considered dysbiotic.

It is impossible to determine the relative significance of dysbiosis in the absence of intestinal microbiota profiles derived from diseased individuals. By sequencing the gastrointestinal microbiota of patients with colon cancer or inflammatory bowel disease, it is often possible to determine the abundance of *E. coli* may be significantly higher than those observed in healthy people. These observations provide associations that necessitate large sample sizes to validate the association's strength. Most dysbioses associated with human disease are not so simple and may involve disturbances in the balance of multiple features of the gut microbiota. A further complication is that the dysbiosis of the gut microbiota associated with a specific disease like type 2 diabetes may not take any single reproducible configuration.

The gut communities in obese subjects, those with type 2 diabetes, Crohn's disease, ulcerative colitis, colorectal cancer, autism-spectrum disorder and many others are dysbiotic. The patterns of dysbiosis are different for each condition and rarely are singular for any specific disease. This complicates the characterization of the dysbiotic communities since they may not be functionally congruent. In fact we know for example in colorectal cancer, different dysbiotic signatures impact the host in distinct ways that are not functionally similar and yet may converge on the end result, promotion of tumors. Such is the nature of complex disease.

Which came first, the chicken or the egg?

Two features common to the diseases we will discuss in Part 2 are microbial dysbiosis and immune dysfunction. We know that microbes, like *E. coli* that produce large quantities of lipopolysaccharide (LPS) can cause inflammation and from this perspective we might conclude that alterations in gut communities precedes and drives immune dysfunction. However, we also know that immune dysfunction and/or elevated inflammation can cause gut dysbiosis, that result in increased abundance of *E. coli*. In the context of human disease, it is often unclear which comes first, perhaps neither does. The connectivity of the gut microbiota and immune system may be wired such that the normal and healthy interactions slowly shift back and forth until a threshold is crossed that we recognize clinically as disease.

Chronic and destructive inflammation.

As we have learned, chronic, low-grade inflammation is a clinical symptom of a wide variety of diseases and reflects the immune system's response to continual encounters with antigens that serve to maintain the immune system in an over- stimulated state. The innate immune system orchestrates the activities of a complex number of immune cell types that seek to rid the body of the offending stimuli through inflammatory processes that facilitate the destruction of harmful microbes, toxins and antigens. These antigens can be from our diet, factors produced by gut microbes, or substances we come into contact within our environment.

The immune system has evolved to defend us from viral and bacterial pathogens, to repair any injury we may sustain, and to attack malignant cancer cells and tumors. These are the most obvious functions of the immune system, given its involvement in numerous other aspects of human physiology, including cognitive, behavioral, and mental disorders. In this regard, it is impossible to overstate the significance of a highly functional and effective immune system in maintaining human health and protecting us from disease.

With this brief overview of the intimate relationship between the gut microbiota and the function of our immune system, we are in a better position to understand the nature of chronic disease and why diet is such an integral part of ensuring that we do not succumb to disease in our lifetime, and why strategies to modulate the gut microbiota through diet, prebiotics, and probiotics discussed in Chapters 14, 15, and 16 offer new promise to alleviate many conditions.

Acting as a consortium, cooperative species are able to assemble the enzymes necessary to assimilate dietary components at the appropriate time and location.

Chapter 7
Antibiotics and the Hygiene Hypothesis.

Germs, germs, everywhere.

Most of us were raised to think of bacteria as "germs" and the source of infection and disease. We were even subtly taught about the main sources of germs, like spoiled food, sneezes and feces. While there is wisdom in these teachings, they unfortunately convey a strong myth at the same time. Bacteria are ubiquitous in our environment. They are literally everywhere. It has been estimated that there are 1×10^{30} bacteria on the planet. This number is well beyond human comprehension, but consider that for every person on the planet, 10 million trillion bacteria exist.

Pathogenic bacteria are extremely uncommon among this staggering number of microorganisms. Thus, the vast majority of microbes are harmless to humans. This should not diminish the power of pathogenic microbes that infect humans and cause disease and even death.

Alexander Fleming's 1928 discovery of penicillin is one of the most significant medical discoveries in history. Several additional antibiotics were discovered in the decades that followed, redefining the global treatment of infectious disease and saving innumerable lives.

Antibiotics: a double edge sword.

Less than one hundred years later, widespread drug-resistance and multi-drug resistant pathogens have rendered some antibiotics practically ineffective. The overuse and misuse of antibiotics in medicine, and even more so in agriculture, now pose a threat to our society, as superbugs that have developed resistance to multiple antibiotics are becoming increasingly prevalent.

Human carnivores contribute significantly to the problem. Estimates of the total use of antibiotics worldwide are highly variable, particularly with regard to the quantity used in the agricultural industry, as surveillance and reporting are inadequate in many nations. The agricultural (livestock) industry uses between 63,000 and 240,000 kilograms of antibiotics annually. Conservatively, the use of antibiotics in the livestock industry is at least equivalent to that of humans. Unfortunately, the overuse of antibiotics creates a strong selective pressure for microbes to develop resistance to these medicines, which they do with remarkable efficiency. Numerous studies have concluded that antibiotic-resistant bacterial genes are transmitted from livestock to humans residing in close proximity to drug-using farms.

The medical al industry's excessive reliance on "last resort" antibiotics used to treat patients with drug-resistant bacterial infections is of particular concern. Utilizing modest doses of antibiotics in livestock for growth promotion is a second hazardous practice. Although it is understandable why livestock producers would employ strategies to promote animal growth, this practice primarily encourages the accumulation of fat mass.

In mice, it has been demonstrated that low-dose antibiotic administration alters the intestinal microbiota rather than virtually eliminating it, leading to increased adipose mass. As alarming as the increased incidence of drug-resistant bacteria is, we now recognize that antibiotics can also alter disease-related human physiology even at sub-therapeutic doses, posing a novel threat to human health.

It would be incorrect to conclude from this information that you should avoid taking antibiotics prescribed by your doctor to treat a bacterial infection. Even for the most astute physician, the responsible use of antibiotics is a formidable challenge. Every parent has likely encountered the situation in which their infant became ill and was susceptible to worsening if not treated promptly. The thought of their child succumbing to an infection is intolerable, causing parents to adopt tunnel vision; they want to ensure their child's health, and physicians are likely to comply, as they too wish for the patient's recovery. In 2010, 74.5 million outpatient children were prescribed antibiotics, which accounted for 25 percent of all prescriptions written for children. The strong desire to keep our children healthy helps to explain this statistic.

The long reach of the gut microbiome.

The use of broad-spectrum antibiotics disrupts the equilibrium of intestinal microbial communities by eliminating significant portions of resident populations, thereby nullifying their collective positive effect on host health. Diarrhea is the most obvious symptom experienced by many individuals taking antibiotics. Antibiotics eradicate a significant portion of the gut microbiota, leaving vacancies in the gut ecosystem. In an ironic twist, this leaves subjects more susceptible to gastrointestinal infections and infections outside of the intestine.

These findings support the gut microbiota's ability to protect us from pathogenic infection, but the fact that this protection extends beyond the gut was much less predictable. For instance, administration of antibiotics that do not permeate the gut and therefore only affect the gut microbiota makes rodents significantly more susceptible to influenza virus lung infection. How does this work?

The protective effect of gut microbiota exemplifies one of the relationships between gut microbiota and immune system discussed in the previous chapter. It also highlights the extensive effects of the gut microbiota on human health that extend beyond gut physiology. It is evident that the signals produced by gut microorganisms influence the gut immune system, which then transmits these signals to distal sites throughout the body, given that the immune system acts throughout our bodies, particularly at environmental boundaries (gut, skin, oral cavity, and lungs).

Several studies have investigated the repopulation of the intestinal microbiota following the completion of an antibiotic course. In general, within a week or so, the previously extant bacterial communities are restored. A few days after the cessation of antibiotics, it is evident that some species exploit the "empty" niche and achieve increased abundance, but over time, the original configuration is restored with remarkable fidelity. Actual microbiota restoration appears to vary from subject to subject and is therefore personalized. Indeed, some people are unable to entirely recover their microbiome after exposure to antibiotics.

The ability to recover.

The ecological term "resilience" refers to the capacity of ecosystems to recover after a perturbation. However, the factors that determine resilience in the context of the intestinal microbiota are not well understood. The resilience of gut microbiota may be a crucial factor in determining susceptibility to dysbiosis and disease; therefore, it is worthwhile to gain a deeper understanding of this phenomenon.

A useful way to visualize the concept of resilience is to imagine a ball that may represent an individual bacterial species or the gut microbiome as a whole. In one person the ball may sit within a trough of a steep hill prior to perturbation, whereas in another individual the ball may sit at the trough of a shallow hill. Finally, in a third individual the ball may sit perched at the peak of a steep hill.

Imagine now that a perturbation is applied to each e.g., diet or antibiotics regimen. In the first individual, the ball may travel up the hill slightly, but will reliably return to its original position once the disturbance subsides. If the perturbation is small enough, the second individual will respond similarly to the first, but if the perturbation is large enough, the ball will travel over the hill and into a new space, never reverting to its original state. Lastly, the third individual is extremely sensitive to any disturbance and prone to dysbiosis if even minor disturbances occur.

Early life events may determine resilience.

This visualization over simplifies the process of microbiome dynamics accounting for stability and resilience but underscores that resilience is personalized. We have learned much about these features of gut microbiota by studying the dynamics of gut microbiota change in newborns over the first year of life. Newborns are born sterile (without any microbiota). Depending on the mode of delivery, the newborn is colonized with distinct microbes. In the case of vaginal deliveries, microbes from the mother's vaginal and fecal microbes are transmitted to the newborn and become the primary colonizers, whereas babies born by Caesarian section are predominately colonized by skin microbes. In other words, our first microbiota is directly determined by our first contacts with the outside world and as we will see, may have impact on the baby's future health landscape.

These pioneer colonizers are inadequately adapted to serve the numerous functions required for an efficient microbiota, but they may play an essential role in establishing a foothold in the gut and other colonized surfaces, thereby preventing pathogens from occupying these niches. The significance of this function stems from its potential compensatory role in the context of an immature newborn's immune system. However, bacteria that ordinarily inhabit the skin cannot perform the specialized functions required in the gut, and vice versa.

Cooperation to establish a utopian microbial community.

As the infant consumes their first meals, well-evolved microorganisms in the breast milk carry out the metabolism of the available milk polysaccharide sugars. These bacteria become the first diet-relevant inhabitants of the gastrointestinal microbiota and establish residence. These bacteria immediately provide a valuable function to break down complex sugars into simpler products that may be assimilated by the newborn. Breast milk is complex and it is likely that the microbes best-suited to facilitate other dietary components such as protein and milk fats also need to be acquired and optimized.

Optimization is a sequential process, and achieving a highly efficient state takes time. Microbes do not perform their functions in isolation; rather, they frequently engage in cooperative interactions with other bacterial species. This is the reason why the process takes so long. All of these cooperative relationships are subject to Darwinian selection, which governs the process of optimization. Cooperation is the best and possibly only way for intestinal bacterial communities to attain sophisticated functional capacity. Compared to their human host, microbial genomes in the intestine encode a small number of genes, limiting the metabolic capacity of individual bacterial species.

Cooperation is the most effective way to maximize the energy and nutrient yield from our diet due to the complexity of the human diet. Complex nutrient degradation is not the responsibility of a single bacterial species, but rather a team effort. Acting as a consortium, cooperative species are able to assemble the enzymes necessary to assimilate dietary components at the appropriate time and location. In this regard, it is possible that the maturation process is one of optimization in which the optimal assortment of species and functional skill sets are assembled.

The gut microbiota endures rapid and significant alterations during the first weeks of life.

Since the diet of newborns is highly controlled, a mono diet of breast milk or formula, the changes in community composition in early life are most likely a reflection of the optimization of functional networks among bacterial species. Interestingly, the rate of change is not constant. In this regard gut microbial communities have a velocity (rate of change) that is very high in the first weeks of life that progressively slows as well adapted communities are assembled.

Here we go again.

When babies begin to eat solid foods to meet their ever-increasing energy demands, the milk-centric microbiota is challenged with new substrates launching another series of adaptations. Once again, the rate of change increases wherein the milk-centric microbiota is replaced by new microbes that are more similar to those commonly observed in adults. New relationships among microbes need to form to optimize the cooperative activities of the community. By the time the baby reaches the age of 1 years old, the gut microbiota possesses greater stability and closely resembles the gut microbiota of an adult. By the age of 2 to 3 years old, the infant microbiome is considered fully matured.

In addition to the inherent interest in understanding how newborn gut microbiomes evolve, knowledge of these processes may have direct bearing on subsequent disease susceptibility. We have learned how the transition from a milk-based to a solid-food diet influences the rate and magnitude of change over time. These results suggest that there is a correlation between the adaptability of gastrointestinal communities and their resistance to perturbation. The developing gut communities appear to be especially vulnerable to perturbations that may reflect the incompleteness of the maturation process that establishes stability through establishment of cooperative microbial networks that have been selected for optimal efficiency and redundancy.

Numerous epidemiological studies have examined whether early-life antibiotic exposure predisposes infants to adult-onset diseases. It is conceivable that the timing of antibiotic exposure has vastly differing effects on the gut microbiome depending on whether or not it is in a state of high flux or nearing a state of high stability. As we have learned, resilience is a characteristic associated with the intensity and number of networks formed within stable "optimized" bacterial communities, and low resilience may be a characteristic of weakly adapted communities that have not formed such networks or has been disrupted one or more times. Consequently, the same perturbation (antibiotic exposure) may have drastically differing effects depending on the status of the gastrointestinal microbiome.

Biodiversity in early life and future health.

We know that both the mode of delivery (vaginal versus Caesarean section) and the infant's diet (breast milk versus formula) influence the overall diversity of the gastrointestinal microbiome. The microbial diversity of caesarean-section-delivered infants is lower than that of vaginally-delivered infants. Similarly, breastfed infants have greater microbial diversity than formula-fed infants. While we do not yet fully comprehend why increased microbial diversity is a desirable attribute, there is ample evidence from other ecological systems indicating that increased biodiversity increases community stability and disease resistance.

Forests composed of a single species are susceptible to being eradicated by a blithe, whereas forests with a high level of species diversity are comparatively resistant to such a blithe. As we know that tall trees provide shade for trees that flourish in low light, the story is more complex than this basic example suggests. Similarly, monoculture farming depletes the soil of the nutrients required by a specific crop, whereas crop rotation replenishes the soil, thereby prolonging the utility of a plot of land. It is probable that microbiota with a high degree of diversity are more resilient because they form more complex and extensive networks of cooperative interactions. These networks may also be fortified with functional redundancy to the extent that the loss of a single species in the community has minimal or no effect on the network's efficiency and function.

We have examined the resilience of gut bacterial communities in the context of functional networks as dictated by dietary harvest efficiency. Its ultimate relationship to human health however, is the dual role of these networks to mediate interactions with the gut immune system. Viewed from this perspective we might think of the inheritance of microbiota at birth and diet are the primary drivers of establishing high-diversity, robustly interconnected microbial communities. These networks must feature bacterial species that engage in positive communication and interactions with the immune system.

The antecedent discussion helps us comprehend the controversial hypothesis that early life exposure to antibiotics has varying effects on future health (disease susceptibility) depending on the timing of exposure. It has been established that specific members of the gut microbiota stimulate complete gut immune development in infants during early life. During this time, the immune system is surveying and familiarizing itself with the healthy intestinal microbiome. This procedure is essential for establishing immune tolerance so that the gut immune system recognizes the gut microbiota as "self"

Epidemiological studies examining infant exposure to antibiotics are inconsistent in some instances, but trends in study conclusions establish associations between early life antibiotic exposure and susceptibility to develop diseases involving immune dysfunction later in life. Some studies have concluded that the body mass index (BMI) of antibiotic-exposed babies younger than six months old increases over time. Although additional research is necessary to confirm these findings, they are consistent with the effects of antibiotics on the adipose mass of livestock and rodents.

Similarly, antibiotic use in the first two years of life is associated with increased incidence of asthma in seven-year-olds. Interestingly, this association was related to the number of antibiotic exposures the infants experienced. The results are strongly mirrored by studies of autoimmune disease, like inflammatory bowel disease (IBD) and others. Children with IBD by the age of 8 were nearly 3 times more likely to have been exposed to antibiotics in the first year of life.

The hygiene hypothesis.

Certain conditions afflicting the millennial generation (those born between 1980 and 1999) have experienced a sharp rise in incidence. The diseases include, among others, atopic disease (asthma, anaphylaxis, food allergy, allergic rhinitis, and dermatitis). In this population, autoimmune diseases such as type 1 diabetes and IBD have also increased. In recent years, the hygiene hypothesis has received considerable attention for its ability to potentially explain the sharp rise in these diseases. The sanitation hypothesis attempts to explain the increased prevalence of disease as a consequence of a reduction in the number of infections, exposure to environmental macro- and microorganisms, and commensal microbiome diversity.

A major component of the hygiene hypothesis is the notion that, as a result of improved hygiene, we have reduced the incidence of infections that, despite being a transient setback to our daily health, serve to safeguard us in the long run by bolstering the robustness of our immune system. Epidemiological analyses demonstrate a correlation between higher socioeconomic status and a higher incidence of autoimmune and allergic diseases. The correlation between hygiene and the incidence of type 1 diabetes suggests that childhood infections may protect against this autoimmune disease.

Infections that have co-evolved with human populations over the millennia are deemed to be more significant, according to the hypothesis. In this respect, two infections have been investigated the most. Hepatitis A virus infections and soil-transmitted parasitic infections such as filariasis, onchocerciasis, and schistosomiasis. In countries with inadequate health care, the prevalence of these infections remains high, while the incidence of allergic disease remains low.

Numerous epidemiological studies have found that decreased family size, urbanization, and increases in affluence may contribute to an increase in immune dysfunction and disease. Moreover, individuals in developed nations are not as frequently exposed to infections by viruses, bacteria, and parasites, thereby altering the development and competence of the immune system to develop and maintain an optimal balance between immune stimulatory pathways and those involved in tolerance. In contrast, the presence of elder siblings, exposure to family pets, and upbringing on a working farm are associated with a lower incidence of allergy and autoimmune diseases such as type 1 diabetes and asthma in adulthood.

Several studies have found that the diversity of intestinal microorganisms in human populations residing in regions that have been minimally impacted by the industrialized world is greater than in the developed world. Although these observations are intriguing, they are difficult to interpret due to the fact that non-industrialized societies differ from industrialized nations with regard to all of the factors believed to mediate the hygiene hypothesis. The popular press has seized upon this correlation, emphasizing that our cultural reliance on antibacterial detergent, cleansing agents, and vaccinations is to blame for the prevalence of disease.

Despite the fact that the hygiene hypothesis appears to be acquiring support as more studies are conducted, the main factors involved are anything but simple for individuals or parents to address. It is essential to remember that antibiotics and vaccines have saved innumerable lives. The possibility that both may have negative effects gives us pause. While data supporting the hygiene hypothesis are accumulating, they are difficult to properly interpret, and much more research is required before we can modify our best decision-making process regarding how to safeguard the health of our children.

Among the thousands of things that have changed as a result of industrialization and urbanization of human populations, it is simply premature to conclude that our increased attention to clean households is placing our children's health at risk. It is not yet possible to define the causal factors with greater precision.

Antibiotic use in childhood may increase disease incidence, but this risk must always be weighed against that of denying antibiotics to children with infections. To reduce the unnecessary administration of antibiotics to treat viral infections, it will be necessary to develop enhanced rapid diagnostic procedures that allow us to distinguish between viral and bacterial infections more swiftly. Similarly, enhanced regulations and guidance regarding the use of antibiotics in the livestock industry should be given significant consideration.

Intentional parasitic infection.

The hygiene hypothesis poses a significant catch-22 situation for everyone. This is extremely unsatisfying; when it comes to safeguarding our loved ones, we prefer answers. How can a parent make satisfactory judgments with this information? Several clinical trials are currently underway to ascertain whether the stimulation of children's immune systems can prevent the development of hypersensitivity and autoimmune diseases in adulthood. The intentional infection of rodents and humans with ova derived from worm parasites such as *Trichuris suis* or *Necator americanus* protects against the development and severity of diseases such as Crohn's disease, according to accumulating evidence.

In Part 3 of the book, we will discuss probiotics in detail; however, probiotics are becoming an increasingly popular method to stimulate the immune system, and there is a large body of evidence supporting their efficacy in the context of antibiotic use. In the context of allergy and autoimmune diseases, probiotics may have a wider spectrum of applications. One of the first examples emerged from studies of expectant women who took *Lactobacillus* GG 2-4 weeks prior to delivery and for 6 months after delivery. This protection lasted up to seven years and reduced the incidence of atopic dermatitis in offspring. Additional research must be conducted in this area because comparable studies have demonstrated fewer or no effects.

In a variety of disease models, the use of bacterial extracts has demonstrated efficacy. Lacking a clear definition of the active components, these extracts may not be readily accepted by the FDA as a treatment method due to the potential for unanticipated risks inherent in ill-defined therapeutics. However, these results do support the notion that the complex antigens produced by the gut microbiota hold potential answers, and that our ability to control diseases in the future using alternatives to broad-spectrum antibiotics may prove to be the most effective way to alleviate this increasing disease burden on our human society.

Part 2
Common Conditions Related to the Microbiome

Our gut microbiota is extremely responsive to the quality of our diet, whether it be healthful or unhealthy.

Chapter 8
Leaky Gut: A Common Thread Amongst Chronic Disease

The term "leaky gut" or intestinal permeability, has only recently entered the popular lexicon, and many who have heard it have only a limited understanding of what it is and, more importantly, the potential health risks it poses. Many clinicians have not yet formally recognized leaky gut as a clinical condition, and there does not appear to be a sense of urgency to recognize this condition in their patients, which can be diagnosed with a simple urine test that measures the extent of leakiness.

What is leaky gut?

To understand what leaky gut is, we must first understand something about the intestinal lining. It is estimated that about 70% of the immune cells in the human body reside in the gut. If we think of the intestine like a tube, we have a massive population of bacteria and food particles on the inside and massive immune cell populations on the outside of the tube. It may therefore be quite surprising that only a single cell layer of intestinal epithelial cells separates these two compartments. The intestinal epithelium must establish a delicate balancing act, that on the one hand allows nutrients to be absorbed while keeping dangerous food antigens and bacteria from doing likewise. Research has established that neighboring cells in contact with one another express proteins that couple and "seal" neighboring cells together. This seal is disrupted in the context of leaky gut.

How important is leaky gut?

Globally, it is estimated that 500 million people are obese and 1.4 billion are overweight. In 1980, 14% of the U.S. population was obese; by 2010, that number had dramatically increased to 35%. Children have been affected disproportionately. During the same time period, the prevalence of childhood obesity (ages 6 to 12) increased from 3.5% to 15% in females and to 20% in boys. In less than four decades, the prevalence of type 2 diabetes increased from 1% to 6% (19 million people) in the United States. Autoimmune disorders, such as IBD, afflict 50 million Americans. A number of extremely debilitating autoimmune disorders disproportionately affect women. Celiac disease is a severe disorder that affects 1% of the global population. This disease is caused by gluten intolerance. It is estimated that 2.5 million Americans are undiagnosed with Celiac disease. Leaky gut, elevated inflammation, and a disruption in the balance of gut bacterial populations, underlie each of these disease epidemics and others.

Multiple lines of evidence indicate that leaky gut may be the underlying cause of these diverse diseases, as overexposure to gastrointestinal contents activates the underlying immune system and causes inflammation. These effects foster a variety of secondary disease manifestations. Therefore, intestinal permeability represents a therapeutic target with enormous potential relevance. Leaky gut is grossly underdiagnosed, and its prevalence cannot be reliably estimated, but it is likely to affect millions in the United States alone. There are no currently available prescription medications or validated treatment methods for leaky intestines.

A clinical gap.

Given what we know about the co-occurrence of leaky gut with a long list of diseases, such as obesity, type 2 diabetes, IBS, autoimmune diseases such as IBD, autism, food allergies such as celiac disease, and others, the failure to recognize leaky gut as an important clinical symptom represents an important gap in clinical practice. In the previous chapter, we learned that the prevalence of these diseases has increased in western populations and other developing nations worldwide over the past several decades. The answers to the question of why leaky gut is a signature of so many seemingly disparate diseases and how leaky gut contributes to these disease states may be revealed by a large number of research studies. We will see the importance of leaky gut as an underlying driving force for the development of these diseases and why the development of preventative measures and treatment strategies represents an urgent undertaking.

Examined individually, the diseases that are increasingly impacting human civilization in recent years appear to be wholly distinct and unrelated to one another. This perception is well-founded, as each of these diseases is extraordinarily complex and, within a single disease, exhibits a great deal of molecular heterogeneity. As we have discussed, the realization that the majority of human diseases, despite being labeled as a single entity, are frequently heterogeneous. This characteristic of disease has inspired the field of personalized medicine, which endeavors to account for the fact that the optimal treatment for an individual afflicted with a common disease is typically not a single intervention.

The search for commonality.

Those invested in treating these diseases, appreciating their complexity, frequently seek to identify the characteristics shared by those afflicted with a particular disease. They do so in order to shed light on the dysregulated pathways, which are alluring therapeutic targets that, if corrected, would restore the entire system to a healthy state. In actuality, such successes are uncommon, as the vast majority of pharmaceutical medications we take do not cure disease but rather modify our physiology to mitigate the effects of dysregulation.

Leaky gut may be a characteristic shared not just by one disease, but by dozens of significant diseases. This may seem like rhetoric, but the more we learn about the causes and effects of leaky intestine, the more plausible this possibility becomes. Examining the intimate relationship between leaky gut, chronic and destructive inflammation, and dybsiosis of the gut microbiome, we will investigate this crucial topic in great depth.

Remarkably, all three of these characteristics are frequently observed in patients suffering from a wide variety of diseases, especially those with a strong environmental component that have increased over the past several decades. We will investigate each of these factors and their interrelationships to determine why they coexist and why they may provide a foundation for curing a variety of diseases in our society.

Gut Microbiota.

We have learned that our gut microbiota is extremely responsive to the quality of our diet, whether it be healthful or unhealthy. Perhaps it is easier to comprehend how an unhealthy diet influences the composition of our gut microbiota and how this influences obesity or gut-related diseases such as food allergies, inflammatory bowel disease, or colon cancer, but what about autoimmune diseases, autism, and other diseases that appear to be independent of the gut microbiota? In fact, each of these diseases are associated with dysbiosis of the intestinal microbiota.

A high-fat diet induces chronic inflammation due to changes in the composition of the intestinal microbiota. Still other dysbioses have the same effect of an increased abundance of pro-inflammatory bacterial species. The question then arises as to whether the prevalence of gut dysbiosis is a significant factor in disease onset or progression or merely a consequence of the disease state itself?

Passenger or driver of leaky gut

Scientists refer to this issue as whether the gut microbiota is a passive passenger or a driver in the disease process. It bears mentioning that it is considerably simpler to establish an association than to establish a disease's causality. The same holds true for intestinal permeability. Is leaky gut simply a manifestation of the improper functioning of independent systems responsible for disease, or does leaky gut set into motion diverse events that account for the wide spectrum of disease that it is associated with?

The frequency with which novel gut microbiota configurations have been reported in association with dozens of diseases over the past several years has led some to develop skepticism and question whether they are all significant. Indeed, scientists are skilled at being skeptical of things that appear too wonderful to be true or too obvious to be real. We simply haven't had enough time to completely address these crucial concerns due to the rapid pace of new discoveries regarding the gut microbiota.

In the cases of obesity and type 2 diabetes, these critical analyses have been performed and help to establish the intestinal microbiota's causative role in disease. Time will reveal the extent of the intestinal microbiota's involvement in disease. In the meantime, there is little evidence to dampen our conviction for the gut microbiota's central role in metabolic and immune disease control.

Gut microbiota dysbiosis, hard to define, hard to see.

With today's powerful sequencing technologies, it is relatively simple to profile the gut microbiota composition of hundreds or thousands of individuals in great detail. By comparing healthy and diseased individuals' gut microbiota profiles, it is also relatively easy to identify distinguishing features in gut microbiota profiles using sophisticated computer algorithms. Such comparisons yield complex results that are typically best described by trends rather than firm and fast principles.

In diseases such as ulcerative colitis, one of the two main pathologies comprising inflammatory bowel disease, numerous individuals exhibit elevated levels of *E. coli* and decreased levels of the anti-inflammatory species *Faecalibacterium prausnitzii*. In addition, microbial communities exhibit a general trend toward decreasing species diversity. The confounding feature of these profiles is that such summaries only describe a subset of humans afflicted with colitis. The gut microbiota of some subjects may fail to present any obvious differences in composition that would be suggestive of disease. Perhaps additional signatures of dysbiosis are present in those individuals?

Subjects with other diseases, such as autism spectrum disorder (ASD), have intestinal microbiota with more complex patterns that are frequently difficult to discern or categorize. Many subjects with ASD may exhibit an "abnormal" microbiota profile, but these abnormalities may be shared by only a small proportion of affected individuals. Why do some diseases result in easily described alterations and others not? Why don't all people afflicted with a particular disease share discrete features of their microbiome? These are the burning questions being addressed by research scientists today who seek to decode the sometimes subtle messages of the gut microbiota.

Autism spectrum disorder, as the name implies, is not a discrete disease and cannot be easily defined by any small set of criteria. Likewise, IBD encompasses two distinct diseases, Crohn's and ulcerative colitis and each of these pathologies similarly lie on a spectrum. The clinical symptomology and molecular aberrancies associated with these diseases are also highly varied across subjects.

Many paths to disease and health restoration.

These results make clear that the improper functioning of numerous host cellular pathways can result in disease. These findings potentially help to explain the diverse range of clinical symptoms presented by patients and why the signatures present in the gut microbiota may not appear uniform. Indeed, it is also likely that the gut microbiota may play a significant role in disease development in some individuals but not others.

Our failure to observe distinct disease signatures in ASD may be due to our inability to properly categorize patients based on the most significant disease characteristics. The problem can be conceptualized as follows. Suppose you had a small notecard and asked fifty individuals to sign it in any location and orientation. As more signatures are added to the card, the individual signatures become less legible, until eventually none of them are recognizable. This may be the primary obstacle preventing improved recognition of microbiome signatures associated with diseases such as ASD; we are simply grouping individuals based on the term autism, obscuring any distinct signatures that may be present. The classical comparison of healthy vs disease individuals is then likely to produce a very blurred signature. If instead, these subjects were sub-classified into 10 distinct disease types, the comparison of gut microbiota profiles of 10 subtypes to healthy controls may be crystal clear.

Similarly, numerous microbiota profiles are generated for individuals with the same disease, but who may have received different treatments. Antibiotics and nonsteroidal anti-inflammatory medications are frequently prescribed for childhood Crohn's disease. In such situations, it becomes challenging to distinguish between intestinal microbiota signatures associated with disease and those that may result from treatment.

In the future, it will be crucial to improve our ability to stratify and classify individuals with complex disease in order to improve our ability to interpret the tea leaves and devise the most effective treatments for disease. To better comprehend this, let's examine the other common characteristics of epidemic diseases.

Chronic low-grade inflammation is a condition between healthy inflammatory tone and acute inflammation. Examining the diseases associated with low-grade chronic inflammation reveals that leaky gut almost always co-exists. An important nuance of leaky gut is that, in theory, even a healthy gut microbiota may be able to drive inflammation, as the immune system will be exposed to elevated concentrations of food and bacterial antigens that signify a danger response in the immune system. Defects in gut permeability may allow the passage of molecules across the gut epithelium that the immune system is not accustomed to "seeing," triggering an immune response to otherwise harmless food antigens.

The integrity of the intestinal barrier is crucial to human health. To completely comprehend the interrelationships between the gut microbiota, inflammation, and leaky gut, it is necessary to investigate what constitutes a strong gut barrier and how it differs from a leaky gut. The integrity of the barrier is determined in part by a group of proteins known as occludin, claudins and zonulin, that serve to create tight seals between adjacent cells. One could think of these proteins as the mortar that seals the gaps between adjacent bricks in a wall. The expression and spatial placement of these proteins is crucial to their ability to create an effective barrier. Unlike mortar, the proper functioning of occludin, claudins and zonulin form pores that stringently permit transit of small molecules such as ions such as sodium between epithelial cells in what is known as the transcellular route.

The epithelial cells lining the gut are not in fact like indistinguishable bricks in a wall but rather contain cells that differentiate into distinct cell types programmed to carry out highly specialized functions. As we learned in chapter 3, one important cell type is goblet cells that generate and secrete mucin proteins into the gut lumen. These proteins become decorated with large clusters of carbohydrates that in the presence of water form a gel structure. The mucin layer creates a physical barrier separating the immune sensitive epithelium from the massive number of microbial cells and food antigens residing in the gut. The mucin layer thickness increases as one travels down the digestive tract in a manner that mirrors the density of bacteria present in those segments, such that the thickest mucin layer is present in the colon where microbial density is the highest.

Still other specialized cells synthesize and secrete anti-microbial peptides that act like antibiotics to prevent microbes from penetrating the protective mucin layer. Finally, immunoglobulins produced by immune cells underlying the epithelium that are secreted into the gut lumen. These immunoglobulins bind to and even coat bacteria and are thought to prevent their ability to breach the epithelium. All of these features contribute to gut barrier function and therefore defects in any of these components can contribute to leaky gut. Indeed, the architecture and number of systems devoted to a strong barrier function make the strongest argument for the importance of leaky gut and begs the question as to why it is not prioritized by the medical community?

Leaky gut, a vicious cycle.

Now we are able to comprehend how and why leaky gut, gut microbiota, and inflammation are interconnected. It is well-established that inflammation has a detrimental effect on the function of proteins that regulate barrier integrity. Defects in the integrity of a barrier expose the immune system to antigens that can cause inflammation. In various contexts, inflammation is known to modify the composition of the gut microbiota and, over time, may select pathogenic species that have evolved mechanisms to flourish in these conditions and contribute to the inflammatory burden.

As you may have surmised, these relationships are at the core of why leaky gut is a serious condition, as the

195

dysfunction of multiple barrier function components can promote leaky gut. Each cog has the ability to influence the function of the others. This is known as a feedback loop in biology. In some maladies, feedback loops can sustain diseased states. Alternatively, feedback loops can help maintain healthy states. This exemplifies why leaky intestine is insidious and should not be ignored.

Feedback loops reinforce health and disease.

The positive feedback loop operating in the context of leaky gut involve the maintenance of an elevated inflammatory state, that promotes and maintains reduced barrier function. A leaky gut further exposes the immune system to microbial and/or dietary antigens. The elevated inflammation often results in alterations in the gut microbiota that select for microbes like *E. coli* that express inflammatory, lipopolysaccharide (LPS) that further induce local and systemic inflammation. LPS is a potent inducer of inflammation and the cause of toxic shock syndrome in extreme cases.

This selection may also favor bacteria that are more pathogenic in nature (opportunistic pathogens) and more invasive, capable of penetrating the gastrointestinal epithelium and coming into direct contact with the immune system, thereby eliciting a robust inflammatory response. In other words, leaky gut is reinforced by gut microbiota and our immune system once it manifests.

Which came first, the chicken or the egg? One might reasonably now ask a question posed in several research studies that attempt to solve the chicken or the egg conundrum. Which component most commonly becomes dysregulated and sets this cycle into motion? The answer to the riddle is not perfectly solved, but it seems that no one thing necessarily goes wrong first, since the dysfunction of any single component is sufficient to promote the cycle. It is known that genetic factors contribute to the incidence of leaky gut, suggesting that individuals have different susceptibilities to developing leaky gut. Epidemiological studies also point to dietary factors as drivers of leaky gut development. We will explore these factors in more detail below.

Caveats that force us to take pause.

Two significant unanswered questions regarding leaky gut are worthy of mention. First, although leaky gut has been linked to a number of diseases and has the potential to promote disease development, it is not yet known whether leaky gut in humans increases disease risk. Second, if the barrier function of diseased individuals were to be restored, would disease symptoms be altered or cured? We do not yet know the answer to either of these queries. The temporal sequence of events has been explored in at least two human diseases, IBD and type 1 diabetes, where both animal and human studies indicate that leaky gut precedes disease onset, strongly suggesting that leaky gut is a root cause driver of disease. There are an increasing number of animal studies demonstrating that restoring intestinal barrier function can positively affect a broad spectrum of physiological and immune states. Despite these convincing studies, leaky intestine in humans has yet to be thoroughly investigated.

Analysis of tissues with documented barrier defects at the microscopic level suggests that the term "leaky gut" may be too general and needs to be quantified. The extent of gaps in the epithelium is typically tiny, differing only slightly from a healthy barrier. The increased permeability may indeed be sufficient to increase the accessibility of small molecules that are ordinarily unable to cross the epithelial barrier. This raises another essential question. How much permeability is required to increase disease susceptibility?

The observed permeability of a permeable intestine is inconsistent with the possibility of bacterial-sized particles penetrating the epithelium. Despite the fact that this observation may be supported by substantial evidence, bacterial translocation across the epithelium (a primary source of inflammation) does increase in frequency in the context of numerous diseases with underlying barrier defects. We may not fully comprehend how gut bacteria circumvent the gastrointestinal barrier, but the existence of this phenomenon is well supported. We still have much to learn about the danger that a permeable intestine poses to human health. On the other hand, the data collected from a variety of animal models strongly support the potential serious health consequences of leaky intestine, particularly in severe cases.

Available diagnostic procedures for leaky intestines should be approached with caution. The most prevalent test of this type is the lactulose/mannitol test, which evaluates the permeability of these carbohydrates based on their presence in a urine sample. These sugars are metabolized by gut microbes present in the colon; consequently, colonic gut barrier defects cannot be reliably measured with this test, whereas it will be a more accurate diagnostic tool for small intestinal barrier defects, such as those commonly observed in patients with ileal Crohn's disease. For identifying colonic barrier defects, such as those observed in ulcerative colitis, the sucralose test may be preferable.

While numerous research studies have identified dietary components associated with or capable of inducing leaky gut in animal models, it remains unclear whether specific dietary components are responsible for leaky gut or whether multiple components contribute to its development. Similarly, we do not yet know how genetic factors that predispose individuals to leaky gut compare to dietary factors. On the basis of epidemiological associations, some dietary components have been examined more thoroughly than others. All of these candidates require additional inquiry, and some have stronger scientific evidence than others.

Emulsifiers, so smooth and creamy.

Among the dietary factors that contribute to leaky gut, one theory that has garnered considerable support implicates high-salt, high-sugar, and high-emulsifier content in certain processed foods. Several studies have investigated the effect that synthetic surfactants and emulsifiers have on the integrity of the intestinal barrier. Emulsifiers are molecules with hydrophilic (water-loving) and hydrophobic (water-hating) groups, similar to lipids.

This chemical property causes these food additives to accumulate and reach even higher concentrations at surface interfaces, such as the mucin layer that provides protection. The mucin layer also contains lipids, predominantly phosphatidylcholine, which forms a hydrophobic barrier at the mucin-lumen interface, limiting the permeability of water-soluble macromolecules. Synthetic surfactants change intestinal permeability in a manner that is not completely understood. Indeed, pharmaceutical companies have conducted the majority of research on emulsifiers since they represent an effective way to increase the absorption of medications into the bloodstream.

Put that packaged pastry down.

The use of emulsifiers as food additives dates back to the 1930s, but the widespread adoption of the Chorley-wood bread process in the 1960s led to a significant increase. This method utilizes emulsifiers to accomplish faster fermentation times, enhanced dough production characteristics, and increased bread shelf life. Currently, it is estimated that over 500,000 tons of emulsifiers are used commercially each year, a figure that continues to rise rapidly. Approximately fifty percent of emulsifier demand is driven by the pastry industry.

Reading labels can be a disorienting experience for the majority of us. The names are challenging to pronounce, and the words have little to no meaning. Common sense dictates that if a food item contains a long list of ingredients that you have never heard of, it is best to avoid eating it. A reliable method and sensible rule of thumb.

To familiarize oneself with the numerous emulsifiers, we can identify recurring themes in their names. For instance, glyceryl 1-monostearate, glyceryl 1-monopalmitate, glyceryl 1-monooleate, and 2-monoglycerides are common food additives, and you should be aware of their presence in the foods you consume and make a concerted effort to reduce your consumption of emulsifier-containing foods. We currently lack sufficient scientific evidence to draw definitive conclusions regarding the effects of synthetic surfactants in the human diet. In this case, there is no incriminating gun, but their ability to increase intestinal permeability indicates that suspicion may be warranted.

Natural treatments for leaky gut

We will now describe a few of the scientific studies that explored the health benefits of various natural substances. There are also formulations for treating leaky gut that are based on scientific observations and are available online. While these formulations may be helpful or even effective in some cases, it is difficult to determine their efficacy due to the lack of large clinical studies that could quantify their relative success in treating leaky intestine. Studies examining the effect of various treatments on the restoration of barrier function defects are provided below.

Many scientific studies indicate that the administration of particular nutrients decreases intestinal permeability. In cell lines, treatment with the amino acids L-glutamine and tryptophan have reduced intestinal permeability. Similar conclusions have been drawn from research on collagen peptides, which are abundant in the amino acids proline, glycine, and glutamine. Interestingly, mineral-rich bone broth contains high concentrations of these three amino acids, which may be one reason for this natural remedy's longevity. Bone broth proponents frequently cite the importance of proline and glycine for tissue development, glycine for the liver and other detoxification pathways, and glutamine for feeding the cells lining the intestines and increasing muscle mass.

In cell culture, Vitamin D, Vitamin A (retinol), and Zinc have also demonstrated efficacy in reducing intestinal permeability. Many polyphenols have shown promise in enhancing gut barrier function, including quercetin (found in red grapes, blueberries and other dark berries, apples, and others), genistein (found in soy), curcumin (found in turmeric), ECGC or epigallocatechin gallate (found in apples, green tea, and blackberries), and kaempferol (found in green tea and numerous fruits and vegetables, including the aforementioned, as well as potatoes, onions, broccoli.

According to *in vitro* data, the essential omega-3 fatty acids DHA or docosahexaenoic acid (found in foods such as algae, fatty fish, fish oil, and in minor quantities in chicken and egg yolks) and EPA or eicosapentaenoic acid (found in algae and fish) can also reduce intestinal permeability. The optimal equilibrium of short chain fatty acids generated by gut microbiota promotes the health of the intestinal lining. On the other hand, studies have shown that consuming trans-fat-rich foods, processed foods, high-sugar foods, foods to which an individual is allergic or sensitive, as well as alcohol, increases intestinal permeability.

We have learned that our gut microbiota is extremely responsive to the quality of our diet, whether it be healthful or unhealthy. Armed with this powerful information and empowered by the powerful effects of our dietary choices on our microbial teammates, we can eat for a healthy gut barrier and include a wide variety of plants and polyphenolics while avoiding alcohol, processed foods, sugar, and trans-fat.

The more we investigate our gut microbiota, the more we conclude that it is a primary regulator of weight gain.

Chapter 9
Obesity and Type 2 Diabetes

In developed nations, the prevalence of a broad spectrum of diseases has increased dramatically over the past several decades. Obesity appears to be the most evident of these disorders. Since 1980, the prevalence of overweight and obese individuals has more than doubled and is projected to reach over 40% of the US population by 2030. There are an estimated 500 million obese persons and 1.4 billion overweight people worldwide. The connection between obesity and more severe diseases such as type 2 diabetes, heart disease, hypertension, stroke, fatty liver disease, osteoarthritis, depression, liver and colorectal cancer, to name a few, is a greater concern from a societal standpoint than the fact that most of us view being overweight or obese as a matter of vanity and low self-esteem.

The practical reality of obesity and its so-called co-morbidities is the anticipated increase in health care costs to treat these individuals, which is projected to exceed $500 billion by 2030. What will happen to our health care system and health insurance costs as a consequence of the obesity epidemic is a crucial concern. Can we as individuals and as a society afford to ignore appropriate education and preventative measures against what appears to be an inevitable increase in obesity rates? Almost undoubtedly, the answer to the second query is no, we cannot. In the 1950s, at the onset of the cold war, the United States established a number of national programs to safeguard our liberties and way of life, including the Presidential physical fitness program. We sought to increase children's exposure to science and technology in an effort to maintain our leadership position in a world that is undergoing swift transformation. When President Kennedy announced to the world that we would send men to the moon, he presented a seemingly insurmountable challenge to the brightest minds from a variety of disciplines. Failure would have been devastating not only to our national pride, but also to our collective belief that anything is possible if we dedicate ourselves to attaining an objective, regardless of its size or difficulty. Is it conceivable that the same nation that rose to the occasion and successfully sent astronauts to the moon cannot defeat the obesity epidemic? The price of failing to fulfill President Kennedy's bold promise that we would land on the moon by the end of the 1960s would have been primarily psychological and political, whereas the price of failing to address obesity may be much more direct, affecting our national economy and the financial security of all taxpayers.

During the Obama administration, the first lady, Michelle Obama, made obesity a priority, endeavoring to raise awareness of the issue, which is the first step in resolving any issue. Although these efforts were commendable, they fell short of addressing the full scope of the crisis, which necessitates a fundamental shift in the foods we consume and our focus on physical fitness. Ignoring these issues virtually ensures that we and our children will become part of the health care problem, robbing us of the opportunity to live a disease-free existence. How can we achieve the necessary change to avoid the dangers of obesity and its associated maladies if our elected officials are beholden to major industries and interests? In an open market economy, we each have a voice based on our individual demands. If our society demands healthful foods, organic produce, and regular exercise, we are able to influence what producers provide. By understanding what a healthy diet is and how to redefine our lives, what we seek, and how we live, we have the ability to profoundly alter not only ourselves but also the world in which we live. In many respects, the required transformation is as significant and challenging as sending a man to the moon. We can reach our goal if we commit as a society to achieving it.

The study of human physiology in the context of obesity has revealed this disease's multi-tissue nature. While it is reasonable to query the necessity of this information, it has resulted in numerous modifications to our simplistic view that weight gain is solely a function of calories consumed versus calories expended. While this remains a useful weight control guideline, we are all aware that merely reducing our daily caloric intake is insufficient to achieve our objectives. By understanding how the functions of our liver, skeletal muscle, adipose tissue (fat), brain, and gastrointestinal tract interact to control an individual's lean muscle to fat mass ratio, we can better comprehend the effects of various dietary supplements that target improved metabolism and function of these tissues. Recent research has identified the microbes residing in our intestines as a significant factor in the obesity equation, thereby expanding the potential for treating obesity and its comorbidities.

Much of what we know about obesity has been gleaned from animal studies, primarily those involving laboratory rodents and rats administered a high-fat diet, which in some cases resembles a typical Western diet. Through such research, we are better able to assess the effects of a high-fat diet on various organ systems. In contrast to other rodent models that do not effectively translate to human physiology, rodent models of obesity appear to be particularly valuable for teaching us how to facilitate weight loss effectively. This chapter examines the current understanding of obesity and how to complement sensible diet and exercise with effective supplements for optimal results.

Chronic low-grade inflammation is an important characteristic of obesity. By producing lipopolysaccharides, which are cell wall components of specific bacteria, the gastrointestinal microbiota can contribute to this inflammation. Some lipopolysaccharides cause inflammation more than others. Specifically inflammatory are the lipopolysaccharides produced by *Escherichia coli*. While some obese human subjects display elevated levels of *E. coli* in their gastrointestinal tract, this is not a consistent finding, whereas elevated lipopolysaccharides in the circulation of obese individuals is a more frequent finding. This raises the question of how the plasma levels of lipopolysaccharide become elevated in subjects who do not appear to have elevated *E. coli* or other organisms that encode inflammatory lipopolysaccharides? This answer most likely reflects an additional common association between obesity and decreased barrier function or intestinal permeability. A common symptom of a variety of diseases, intestinal permeability or leaky gut allows substances that are typically regulated or prohibited to travel through or around the intestinal wall. In this regard, despite the prevalence of *E. coli* is not enhanced, the inflammatory effect of their lipopolysaccharide can still have a deleterious impact on the host.

A system operating in the gut that involves the function of L cells that represent the enteroendocrine system may play a dominant role in sensing the signals generated by the gut microbiota that influence a number of aspects of obesity, such as leaky gut, satiety, liver steatosis, brown fat thermogenesis, skeletal muscle and white adipose tissue inflammation. In what is known as a positive feedback loop, when this system is stimulated by lipopolysaccharides and other microbial antigens, host cell membrane lipids present in adipose tissue act as signaling molecules that reduce gut barrier function and reinforce the exposure to these offending antigens. Inflammation has numerous negative effects, but in relation to obesity, it causes insulin resistance. This will be discussed in greater depth below. *Akkermansia muciniphila*, a previously mentioned species with extremely low abundance in obese subjects and substantially elevated abundance in slender individuals, has been shown to positively modulate the activity of the enteroendocrine system, which is an intriguing finding. The administration of *A. muciniphila* to rodents as a probiotic, improved barrier function and decreased blood levels of inflammatory lipopolysaccharide.

In many regards, *A. muciniphila* has many characteristics of an outstanding probiotic for treating obesity and type

2 diabetes, but it only recently was deemed by the FDA as generally regarded as safe or GRAS. The GRAS probiotic species are comprised primarily of *Bifidobacterium* and *Lactobacillus* species, which, due to their presence in foods ingested for decades without known adverse health effects, have been grandfathered as probiotics that do not require FDA approval for use. Studies of the microbiome have revealed an assortment of additional species that show promise as an effective probiotic to treat a variety of diseases; however, for these probiotics to be FDA-approved, expensive clinical trials that are just as rigorous as those required for the approval of new pharmaceutical drugs will be necessary. Consumers who favor the use of natural remedies to help manage disease may find this conservative stance on new probiotics frustrating, but there are alternatives of interest. For instance, the prebiotic inulin promotes the proliferation of *A. muciniphila*, potentially rendering the probiotic unnecessary. Large human intervention studies have not yet established the efficacy and uniformity of responsiveness to inulin treatment, but there is a strong likelihood that in the near future prebiotic products will become increasingly accessible as an integrative treatment for disease.

The resulting increase in systemic inflammation has negative effects on multiple tissues, resulting in an increase in fatty liver (steatosis) and a reduction in energy expenditure. It is estimated that 20% of daily energy expenditure is attributable to brown fat activity, a process known as thermogenesis that produces heat and is used by all warm-blooded animals to regulate body temperature. Thyroid hormones of the sympathetic nervous system, such as norepinephrine and leptin, regulate thermogenesis. Intriguingly, it is known that the gastrointestinal microbiota regulates leptin production in one of the numerous ways it communicates with the hypothalamus. Leptin is a hormone that signals when we are satiated and should cease eating. The insensitivity of some obese subjects to the action of leptin establishes a distinct link between overeating and obesity. These associations have led to the realization that altering the composition of the gastrointestinal microbiota may be an effective method to increase brown fat thermogenesis, thereby increasing energy expenditure and decreasing adiposity in obese people. For instance, guar gum, a prebiotic compound, and green tea, both of which have demonstrated anti-obesity effects, stimulate brown fat thermogenesis. Thermogenic exercise supplements are also intended to stimulate brown fat thermogenesis; however, these supplements have not been thoroughly studied to identify any potential adverse side effects.

Leptin is regarded as the primary regulator of adiposity; therefore, it merits further discussion. Mice lacking the gene encoding leptin gorge themselves and become obese. This activity is opposed by the hunger-inducing hormone ghrelin, which sends signals to the brain. These hormones serve a specific function in the evolution of mammals, and in prehistoric times when food was limited, humans benefited from their ability to regulate energy stores and expenditures. In the majority of developed nations, energy is no longer limited and is therefore overconsumed. In this regard, the system designed to maintain energy balance in times of scarcity serves a counterproductive function when we routinely excessively eat and reduce our sensitivity to the hormone leptin. When we are frequently famished or deprived of food, our fat mass decreases and we produce less leptin, which signals us to consume more and store fat, whereas when we overeat, leptin levels rise, indicating that we have had enough. Since leptin is produced by adipose cells, obese individuals produce more leptin to aid in reducing daily caloric intake; however, obesity circumvents this negative feedback loop. While obese individuals do produce more leptin, the brain's insensitivity to leptin prevents the signal to cease eating from being correctly perceived, resulting in overeating and a vicious cycle.

As previously stated, obesity is significantly linked to type 2 adult-onset diabetes. The more we investigate our gut microbiota, the more we conclude that it is a primary regulator of weight gain. We observe how specific groups of microorganisms influence our cholesterol level, specifically the amount of healthful cholesterol known as high-density lipids (HDL). Similar to the function of glucose tolerance and insulin sensitivity in modulating type 2 diabetes, the role of the gut microbiome may play a significant role in the regulation of type 2 diabetes-related aspects such as glucose tolerance and insulin sensitivity. Similar to type 1 diabetes, the pancreas that produces insulin and regulates glucose homeostasis is dysfunctional. Type 1 diabetes is an autoimmune disease in which insulin-producing islet cells in the pancreas are attacked by the immune system, resulting in an insulin deficiency. Insulin may be produced at normal concentrations in type 2 diabetes, but cells unable to sense insulin due to decreased expression of the protein receptor that binds to and detects circulating insulin levels. Insulin insensitivity is an essential clinical parameter of type 2 diabetes, which is described by this phenomenon.

The inability to correctly regulate glucose levels due to insulin dysregulation is the second essential clinical parameter of type 2 diabetes, glucose insensitivity. Insulin resistance is more likely to develop in individuals who consume a diet elevated in fat. This fact serves to explain the significant relationship between adiposity and type 2 diabetes. This connection is also evident in the composition of the gastrointestinal microbiota, as certain species associated with obesity characteristics such as adipose mass and leptin production are also linked to glucose tolerance and insulin sensitivity. As we have learned, the robust microbiota modulatory activity of our diets enables us to see a fairly comprehensive picture of the interdependence between obesity and type 2 diabetes.

While there are numerous efforts to develop pharmaceuticals that target key regulators of obesity and type 2 diabetes for the treatment of these epidemic diseases, these efforts have not yet been fully realized. With the recent identification of the intestinal microbiota as a factor controlling these diseases, a number of studies are focusing on identifying effective compounds and dietary supplements to treat these conditions. Numerous studies strongly support the ability of certain compounds to prevent weight gain and the associated insulin resistance caused by a high-fat diet. These natural therapeutics are a potent alternative to pharmaceuticals that may cause unwanted side effects and do not address the fundamental cause of the problem. For instance, if we envision a perfect treatment that corrects insulin insensitivity in type 2 diabetics, it is unlikely to correct the chronic inflammation, fatty liver, or cardiovascular disease risk associated with a Western diet. In this regard, natural therapies that target the intestinal microbiota may be side-effect-free and address the underlying cause of these debilitating diseases.

Ganoderma lucidum has been demonstrated to be an attractive example of a natural therapy (mushroom) for the treatment of obesity and type 2 diabetes. This traditional Chinese medicine has been used for centuries to promote health and longevity, but its potential to reduce diet-induced obesity in rodents has only recently been evaluated. Mice fed a high-fat diet gained weight and fat mass, whereas animals given a solution containing 8 mg of mushroom extract lost weight and fat mass. This is equivalent to a dose of approximately 20 grams for a 150-pound individual. The extract of mushrooms decreased the diameter and size of adipose cells. When our volume increases as a result of obesity, it is primarily due to an increase in fat cell size, not an increase in the number of fat cells. Additionally, the treatment decreased the quantity of adipose deposition in the liver. The most significant effect was the significant decrease in systemic lipopolysaccharides and other markers of inflammation associated with obesity.

Mushroom extract altered the composition of the intestinal microbiota, restoring the levels of certain species that were directly impacted by a high-fat diet to their original levels as measured on a normal low-fat diet. Ganoderma lucidum contains a polysaccharide that mimics the effects of mushroom extract, suggesting that its effects are mediated by a prebiotic mechanism. This mushroom, which is commercially available, has not yet been evaluated in human trials; however, the majority of what we have learned using rodent models of obesity translates effectively to humans, suggesting its potential as an anti-obesity treatment. This example illustrates the nature of prebiotic therapies that function by altering the microbiota of the gut. While the mushroom extract had a significant impact on reducing inflammation, its effect on adiposity and weight gain was rather modest. While this does not diminish the therapeutic potential of Ganoderma lucidum, it does emphasize the complexity of disease and the difficulties inherent in reversing the negative effects of a high-fat diet.

We learned about polyphenolic compounds and nutraceuticals in a previous chapter. For example, black currant seeds contain an abundance of polyphenols, vitamin C, and pectin, a likely prebiotic. When given to rodents fed a high-fat diet, black currant had a negligible effect on weight gain but a greater effect on blood glucose and glucose tolerance. The effect of quercetin and resveratrol on rodents fed a high-fat, high-sugar diet was more impressive. Quercetin altered the composition of the gastrointestinal microbiota more effectively than resveratrol or the combination of the two. The same outcomes were observed in terms of *Akkermansia muciniphila* abundance. Resveratrol had the greatest effect on the expression of tight junction proteins, which are responsible for creating tight closures in the gut epithelium and enhancing gut barrier function. The effects of polyphenolic compounds are consistent with their anti-oxidant and anti-inflammatory properties and demonstrate, once again, that reducing inflammation alone is not enough to substantially reduce weight gain, despite its importance. These results support previous assertions regarding the difficulty of a single compound reversing all of the negative physiological aspects of obesity and type 2 diabetes, but they also begin to reveal which combinations of compounds may be most effective at doing so.

Collectively, these findings suggest that the gastrointestinal microbiota play a significant role not only in the regulation of tumor growth, but also in the overall sensitivity to checkpoint inhibitor therapy.

Chapter 10
Cancer and the Gut Microbiome

The war on cancer, are we winning or losing?

We have declared war on cancer, a conflict that has been ongoing since the Nixon administration. Significant progress has been made in our understanding of how and why cancer develops. Numerous research studies have elucidated the changes that occur in cells as they transform from normal to malignant. With each passing decade, new cancer research topics emerge that hold promise for the long-sought cure, but the solutions remain elusive, and disappointment and failure become more of an expectation than a surprise. A growing number of individuals are demanding explanations as to why the cure is not yet available. Others, who are more susceptible to conspiracy theories, believe that there is a cure for cancer, but that pharmaceutical companies are concealing it because they make more money treating cancer than curing it.

So why haven't scientists yet developed a cure? The simple answer is that cancer is extremely complex. Despite the fact that malignancies share some common features, their underlying causes are not uniform. Cancer development is a multistep process involving random or inherited gene mutations that predispose cells to malignancy. These early precancerous stages appear random, but they can be influenced by a variety of environmental factors, including diet, contaminants and pollutants, age, and others. The majority of accumulated mutations in cells are neutral, while others may signal for the annihilation or mortality of cells carrying the mutation. Some mutations contribute more to the development of cancer than others. Loss of function of tumor suppressor genes can result in profound changes in the rate of additional mutations and/or the cell's capacity to maintain genome integrity. Simply put, cancers involve the breakdown of multiple pathways and cellular functions. In this regard, drug developers routinely test new drugs that target these pathways and often accomplish precisely what was intended only to realize that cancer persists. The challenge facing biomedical research is to identify the "Achilles heel" of cancerous cells that when corrected is sufficient to cure the disease.

The complexity of cancer revealed.

The complexity and non-uniformity of events leading to cancers are the fundamental reason why they are so difficult to treat. The loss of DNA gene functions involved in DNA repair, the inability to correct mutations as they form, or functions that maintain chromosome stability results in enormous changes not only in the number of mutations that accumulate but also in the number of copies of genes present on chromosomes. Whereas normal cells contain two copies of each chromosome, one maternally and one paternally inherited, each encoding individual genes as pairs, cancerous cells undergo both deletions and so-called gene amplification events that can impact many contiguous genes as they appear on one or the other chromosomal copy. In some instances, genes that are normally present in two copies per cell may become amplified to the point where tens or even hundreds of copies exist.

When specific regions containing genes involved in the cell cycle or those regulating cell division are altered, cells are able to disregard normal cues and begin to divide uncontrollably and rapidly. This phenomenon is known as chromosome instability, and it is characteristic of the majority of cancers. Chromosomal instability is random, but given enough events and abnormalities, cancer-promoting genes will eventually be affected. It is crucial to recognize that malignant cells retain the characteristics of chromosome instability. As cancer cells divide, the likelihood that subsequent cancer cells will begin to exhibit gene mutations, gene loss, and amplified gene regions increases. The unfortunate result of this series of events is the formation of a tumor that has an enormous heterogeneity. Moreover, these events are not identical in any two individuals, therefore a new therapy may work perfectly for one individual but not at all for ten others. While these realities paint a dismal picture and would seem to indicate a lack of hope for finding a cure, research efforts continue and are now seeing substantial promise from strategies that boost our body's immune system to attack cancerous cells and eliminate them. Interestingly, these strategies success require certain gut microbes to be present and others to be absent.

The challenges of treating cancer.

The heterogeneity of tumor cells has significant implications for both the study and treatment of cancer, and explains why, despite decades of intensive research, we still lack cures. Any conceivable treatment, based on the best available research and testing, may have dramatic effects on the majority of tumor cells, but due to the enormous heterogeneity of tumor cells, it may at some point hit a significant roadblock, a group of cells that do not respond and can now take over as the "treatment resistant" tumor cells recover from the insults of the therapy. This is one of the most insidious features of cancer. Oncologists are acutely aware that even the most effective antitumor medications are only as effective as the rate at which drug resistance develops. The disheartening process that so many families have witnessed involving loved ones who initially responded well to chemotherapy only to eventually develop resistance to treatment is all too familiar. The development of drug resistance in cancer is very similar to the development of antibiotic resistance in bacterial cells. Given sufficient mutations and alterations in gene function, there is a probability that tumor cells will acquire mutations that render them resistant to chemotherapy.

This description of cancer development, while accurate, is necessarily an over simplification that neglects other aspects and mechanisms whereby cells ultimately divide in an uncontrolled manner. As a means of controlling tumor growth, the earliest chemotherapeutic medications, some of which are unfortunately still in use, targeted the property of uncontrolled cell division. These chemotherapies are not magical; they were merely toxic substances that affected actively dividing cells preferentially. While many chemotherapeutic treatments are effective in controlling tumor growth, the well-known side effects of cancer treatment arise because other cells in the body also are dividing, albeit not at nearly the same rate as tumors.

A major conceptual breakthrough.

With this information, we are now in a position to comprehend a long-standing query in cancer research. The gene mutations and loss of chromosome stability produce genes encoding proteins that are absent from normal human cells. Neo-antigens are the name given to these tumor-specific proteins because they are newly generated during malignancy. In chapter 6, we learned that the immune system responds to pathogenic infections by recognizing foreign (not self) antigens. In addition, we discovered that in the majority of cases, the immune system aggressively attacks and eradicates such infections. Why aren't cancer cells presenting neoantigens to the immune system similarly attacked and eradicated?

Recently, an answer to this question has been provided. We now know that tumor cells produce signals that inhibit the immune system from performing its intended function, which is to attack and eradicate foreign objects. This realization led to a flurry of efforts to determine how tumors were able to inhibit immune attack. Tumors express proteins named immune checkpoint proteins. Expression of these checkpoint proteins neutralize immune cells by tricking the immune system into seeing the tumor as "self," resulting in a tolerance response and suppression of destruction functions.

A new buzz over checkpoint inhibitors.

This understanding has resulted in a significant breakthrough in cancer research and a new class of cancer therapies. Scientists have developed checkpoint-specific antibodies that, when bound to tumor cells, inhibit their capacity to suppress immune attack. These antibodies are known as checkpoint inhibitors. For example, the FDA has approved the use of two checkpoint inhibitors (Ipilimumab and Atezolizumab) to treat melanoma, certain varieties of lung cancer and others. Some patients with malignancies with extremely high mortality rates are cured by these treatments, demonstrating their remarkable effectiveness. It is estimated that only 10 to 20% of individuals respond to these treatments. As a result, the game of chess continues as researchers focus on determining why some patients respond excellently to checkpoint inhibitor therapy while others do not.

An enormous surprise.

Unexpectedly, the variation in the composition of gastrointestinal microbiota may account, at least in part, for the differences in response to checkpoint inhibitor therapy. This result was first demonstrated by the observation that two genetically identical mouse lines obtained from different vendors exhibited distinct tumor growth control in a model of melanoma. Jackson

Laboratories (JAX) mice exhibited slow-growing tumors, whereas Taconic (TAC) mice exhibited rapid tumor growth. Importantly, this model used healthy mice wherein tumor cells were injected subcutaneously into mice to allow tumor formation. Since these rodents were genetically similar and otherwise healthy, it was reasoned that the difference in tumor growth must be due to an unidentified environmental factor.

This hypothesis prompted the researchers to question whether the different gut microbiota in these rodents held the answer. Indeed, when directly compared, the intestinal microbiota of these rodents was distinct. By introducing JAX mouse faeces into TAC mice (a form of fecal microbiome transplantation, aka FMT), it was clearly demonstrated that this difference was responsible for the behavior of tumor growth. The transplantation of JAX faeces into TAC mice produced tumors with growth rates comparable to those observed in JAX mice. The probiotic species *Bifidobacterium longum* was tested as a potential mediator of the slowed growth of tumors after a more thorough examination of the gastrointestinal microbiota present in JAX mice.

When *B. longum* was administered to TAC mice, tumor growth was significantly suppressed, similar to what was observed in JAX mice. Interestingly, treatment of TAC rodents with *B. longum* and the checkpoint inhibitor Atezolizumab, tumor growth was inhibited in a manner that was additive. Collectively, these findings suggest that the gastrointestinal microbiota play a significant role not only in the regulation of tumor growth, but also in the overall sensitivity to checkpoint inhibitor therapy. This seminal research marked a significant advancement in cancer therapy while shedding light on the gut microbiota as a critical factor modulating tumor growth.

The immediate question that surfaced was how the gut microbiota could influence distal melanoma tumors. This query was answered in the same study that demonstrated that gut microorganisms interact with the gut immune system to activate immune cell populations, which then migrate to the site of tumors to enhance their anti-tumor capacity. Collectively, these findings suggest that probiotics and/or FMT may be an effective means of enhancing the uniformity and overall response to checkpoint inhibitor therapies. Caution must be applied here since it remains to be shown that these promising observations made in mouse models of melanoma apply to human cancers. There is little doubt that such research is being actively pursued and that results will be forthcoming.

More than one way to destroy a tumor.

While melanoma tumors were efficiently controlled by Ipilimumab treatment in rodents, this effect was not observed in germ-free mice lacking a microbiome. In accordance with this finding, when conventional mice were treated with antibiotics to eradicate the gut microbiota, the efficacy of Ipilimumab decreased. Immune interactions with closely related species *Bacteroides thetaiotaomicron* and *Bacteroides fragilis* were associated with Ipilimumab therapy responsiveness in both mice and humans, suggesting that these species may mediate the antitumor effects of this checkpoint inhibitor. Interestingly, *B. fragilis* had previously been shown to regulate immune cells via *B. fragilis'* production of the polysaccharide known as PSA. When either *B. fragilis* or PSA was introduced orally into germ-free mice, treatment restored Ipilimumab tumor inhibition.

Liver cancers and the duality of gut microbiota.

The etiology of liver cancers is diverse and can arise due to viral infection, chronic exposure to toxic chemicals, diet and others. The high fat western diet has been directly associated with the growing obesity and type 2 diabetes epidemic in the US and many other developed and developing countries worldwide. Obesity has been linked to an increased risk of developing liver disease and cancer. Given what we learned in Chapter 9 about the connection between the gut microbiota and obesity, it seems reasonable to investigate the gut microbiota as a factor in obesity-induced liver cancer.

A study examining the intestinal microbiota of both genetically and high-fat diet-induced obese rodents that develop liver cancer was recently published. The genetically obese mouse lacks the gene encoding leptin, a hormone that regulates appetite (satiety), resulting in rodents that overeat and become obese as a consequence of an increase in caloric intake. Both obesity models in mice modify the composition of the intestinal microbiota. The increased abundance of bacterial species that metabolize liver-produced bile acids and generate the bile acid deoxycholic acid (DCA) is shared by both microbial communities.

DCA is mutagenic (can cause mutations) and induces the production of pro-inflammatory and tumor-promoting signals and factors. When these mice were treated with a carcinogenic compound to induce liver cancer, genetically obese and high-fat diet-induced obese mice had a greater number of tumors than normal-weight mice. Consistent with this finding, the number of liver tumors was significantly reduced in obese rodents treated with antibiotics to diminish intestinal microbes. In this context, it is clear that gut microbes present in obese mice played the role of villain, promoting liver cancer.

In another model of liver cancer, cells derived from liver tumors are subcutaneously injected into mice where cisplatin (a chemotherapeutic drug) and a probiotic bacteria mixture were compared. Cisplatin targets actively proliferating cells, and while it is notably effective at inhibiting the growth of liver tumors (hepatocellular carcinoma), it is also highly toxic. *E. coli* is found in the probiotic used in this investigation. A commercially available probiotic mixture containing *E. coli* Nissle 1917, *Lactobacillus rhamnosus* GG, and heat-killed VSL#3.

This probiotic, when administered prior to or simultaneously with tumor cell injection, partially inhibited tumor growth, although not to the same degree as cisplatin. A decrease in an immune cell type that mediates inflammation and functions required for angiogenesis, a term characterizing blood vessel formation and vascularization required to sustain high tumor growth rates, is the mechanism by which probiotics exert their anti-tumor effects.

These findings support the ability of the gut microbiota to alter immune cell activities at distant sites and demonstrate how these effects influence processes such as angiogenesis, a critical determinant of tumor growth due to the fact that actively dividing tumor cells have very high metabolic demands and require blood-derived energy to support their growth. While the preventative potential of this probiotic to reduce tumor growth was evident in this mouse model, it has yet to be validated in human liver cancer, where it would most likely be administered to patients with preexisting liver cancer. The inclusion of optimized probiotic formulations could enable clinicians to effectively treat liver cancers with lower doses of cisplatin, thereby reducing the toxicity patients experience during treatment.

Colorectal cancer.

On the basis of a number of indirect lines of evidence, the connection between the intestinal microbiota and colon cancer was one of the first to be examined. For instance, the incidence of intestinal cancers correlates with the density of bacteria, which, as we have learned, is lowest in the first portion of the small intestine (duodenum) and increases by several factors of ten in the final portion of the small intestine (ileum) and even more dramatically in the large intestine (colon). The incidence of colon cancer is 12 times higher than that of small intestine cancer. Germ-free mice develop significantly fewer colon malignancies than conventional mice with endogenous microbiota. Human subjects with IBD and dysbiosis of the intestinal microbiota are five times more likely to develop colon cancer.

These observations prompted a series of investigations investigating the association between gut microbiota community composition in physical proximity to tumors in subjects with colon cancer. Several studies confirmed that gut microbiota composition is strongly altered.

Several distinct dysbioses are observed including sharp increases in *E. coli* in some cases and/or *Fusobacterium nucleatum* a bacterium normally present only in the oral cavity. These studies were unable to determine whether the increased abundance of these species was a result of the bacteria's role in promoting tumor formation or a result of the growth advantage conferred by tumors to these bacteria.

According to a comprehensive analysis of these bacterial species, both promote tumor formation in distinct ways. The *E. coli* involved in colon tumorigenesis is a strain with a distinct set of genes not found in other *E. coli*. Several of these gene sequences are necessary for the production of a toxin that can induce mutations in host cells. As we have learned, *E. coli* is also capable of inducing inflammation through the production of lipopolysaccharide. Interestingly, colonizing germ-free mice with toxin-producing *E. coli* and *Enterococcus faecalis* both caused comparable levels of inflammation in recipient mice, however only *E. coli* induced tumors, suggesting that inflammation is necessary but not sufficient to drive intestinal tumors and that *E. coli* toxin production in combination with host inflammation efficiently promotes tumor formation.

Detailed studies focused on *F. nucleatum* have demonstrated that this bacterium promotes intestinal tumors in rodents *via* mechanisms independent of

236

inflammation, distinguishing it from how *E. coli* causes tumor growth. Two distinct mechanisms have been identified by which *F. nucleatum* promotes the formation of tumors. In the initial, *F. nucleatum* interacts physically with natural killer cells, a crucial anti-tumor immune cell type. This interaction inhibits the normal activity of these cells to assault malignancies. Additionally, it has been established that *F. nucleatum* secretes short proteins (peptides) that inhibit anti-tumor immune responses.

Regarding gut microbiota, the relationship between intestinal and non-intestinal malignancies reveals an unexpected dichotomy. The microbiota of non-intestinal cancers does not drive blooms of pathogenic bacteria but rather involve the lack of "healthy" microbes that positively stimulate the immune system's anti-tumorigenic activities. By contrast, intestinal cancers seem to feature pathogenic microbes that contribute to cancer development and/or progression. This distinction is most clearly seen in experiments involving antibiotic treatment of tumor bearing mice. The ablation of the gut microbiota with antibiotics reduces tumor burden in intestinal cancers but increases it in distal cancers.

This distinction is intriguing, but its practical significance is unclear. It is unknown whether probiotic and microbiome-based therapies, which show such promising results in treating distal tumors, will be effective or ineffective in treating intestinal cancers. The compelling evidence that the gastrointestinal microbiota promotes anti-tumor properties in response to distal tumors will undoubtedly inspire comparable research on colon cancer.

It is noteworthy that while microbial therapeutics for treatment of colon cancer remain unclear, the dysbiosis associated with pre-malignant and malignant colon cancers are fueling powerful diagnostic developments. It is likely that simple stool tests that measure the abundance of individual species present in gut communities can predict your health status or the presence of non-malignant polyps or malignant cancer in individuals. The ability of these tests to identify pre-malignant conditions is exciting and may represent a significant component of cancer prevention in the near future.

A marriage made in heaven.

One of the unanticipated outcomes of these findings is the merging of two of the most potent anti-cancer forces. Cancer biologists and immunologists pursued separate scientific endeavors for many years. They spoke different languages and regarded their interests to be mainly dissimilar. While it had been acknowledged that the immune system played a significant role in controlling tumor growth, the immune system's general inability to do so diminished the value of immunologists in the fight against cancer. This division has been eliminated and a unified front has been firmly established, drawing together some of the brightest minds in science to address one of the most difficult problems in biology and human health.

New frontiers in our understanding of gut microbes.

In a relatively brief period of time, the gut microbiota has risen to the forefront of cancer research. Recent discoveries have illuminated the possibility of altering gut microbiota using probiotic, prebiotic or FMT-based strategies in order to increase the number of people who respond favorably to checkpoint inhibitors or conventional chemotherapy, as well as the potency of that response. It will be essential to conduct parallel studies to enhance our capacity to deliver large quantities of active probiotics to their site of action. Encapsulation technologies appear to hold great promise in this regard, as they appear capable of shielding probiotic bacteria from the harmful effects of gastric acid and releasing bacteria at the desired time, as the probiotic reaches the small or large intestine.

Our enhanced academic understanding of how microbiota induce pro- and anti-tumor responses suggests that our resident gut microorganisms may be considered an extension or newly discovered arm of the human immune system. The two-way communication between the gut microbiota and the immune system positions the gut microbe as both being directed by the immune system and also dictating the status of the immune system throughout the body.

It is difficult not to be amazed by the rapid evolution of the human perception of excrement. Numerous component species of the gut microbiota have the potential to function as drugs of the next generation. The true beauty of achieving this potential lies in the fact that these drugs are natural and devoid of the deleterious adverse effects associated with conventional drugs. It is entirely conceivable that in coming decades, widespread use of microbiome-based therapies for disease prevention and treatment will significantly contribute to a new revolution in human health. Indeed, exciting times have dawned.

While some technical and translational limitations must be overcome, the current mechanistic insights show promise for the emergence of highly efficacious psychobiotics and the targeted, therapeutic modulation of the gut-brain axis in the near future.

Chapter 11
The Microbiota-Gut-Brain Axis: Who is the Puppet Master?

As scientific discoveries are made, medicine in turn continues to evolve. It was once thought that the brain was the "command center" of the body. Now we know that communication in the body is complex and widespread. The communication between the microbiota, gut, and brain is referred to as the microbiota-gut-brain axis or simply the gut-brain axis. This communication occurs in various ways and with various players. Neither the brain nor the gut microbiota is truly the 'puppet master'. The elegant communication is a complex dance with either partner taking the lead and at other times a balance of steps being performed.

Gut-brain axis.

The gut-brain axis refers to interactions between the enteric nervous system in the gastrointestinal (GI) tract and the central nervous system via a bi-directional communication system composed of neural (the "hard wiring") and humoral (endocrine, immunologic, nutritional signals, and other molecules free floating in the milieu) pathways that influence brain function and behavior. The enteric nervous system, also known as the "second brain", contains as many nerves as the spinal cord, regulates fundamental gut functions such as gut motility, intestinal permeability, secretion, and mucosal immune activity, and shares similar neurotransmitters and signaling molecules with the brain. In addition to gastrointestinal functions, the gut microbiota affects critical functions associated with mood, behavior, pain, and cognition.

The gut-brain axis now includes the microbiota as a crucial component. In addition, disturbances in the microbiota-gut-brain axis have been associated with a variety of immune-related, neurological, gastrointestinal, and psychiatric disorders. Alterations in gut-brain signaling are also linked to gut inflammation, abdominal pain, eating disorders, and modifications in healthy stress responses and behavior. In gastrointestinal diseases such as irritable bowel syndrome (IBS) and inflammatory bowel disease (IBD), for instance, there is a high co-occurrence of stress response-related symptoms such as anxiety and depression, highlighting the significance of this axis in the pathology. Connecting the gut microbiota, microbe-derived metabolites, nervous system, and immune system, the complex network of communication regulates processes ranging from gastrointestinal homeostasis to cognitive functions. Consequently, therapeutic modulation of this axis represents a prospective target for the reduction of a number of disorders, including obesity, pain syndromes, psychiatric disorders, and gastrointestinal diseases such as IBS and IBD.

Gut-brain signaling.

The brain communicates with the GI tract via multiple, parallel neural circuits that include both the sympathetic (fight or flight functions) and parasympathetic (rest and digest functions) two divisions of the autonomic nervous system, which regulates basic physiological processes, as well as the hypothalamic-pituitary-adrenal axis (HPA), which is crucial for the regulation of stress responses. Due to unique anatomical features, peripheral metabolic signals, such as nutrients and hormones, can circulate in the bloodstream and access one region of the hypothalamus without traversing the blood-brain barrier. An additional intriguing region of the hypothalamus contains neurons with receptors for the sugar glucose and the hunger hormone leptin, as well as the brain-derived neurotrophic factor (BDNF), a satiety/anorexic neuropeptide. Leptin, a hunger hormone, is produced by fat cells and enteroendocrine cells lining the gut, and its concentrations in systemic circulation are proportional to body fat mass. Leptin receptors are highly expressed in the hypothalamus, and activation of leptin signaling results in decreased food intake and increased energy expenditure. Insulin, an additional adiposity marker, contacts receptors in the hypothalamus, thereby transmitting a signal of satiety to the brain. Another region involved in nutrition behavior and energy balance is the medulla. The sensory vagus nerve transmits satiety signals to the solitary tract nucleus in the medulla oblongata, which receives both humoral and neural signals. Consequently, peripheral metabolic signals and nutrients communicate with the brain via the hypothalamus, medulla, and certain regions of the midbrain.

The gut has been recognized as the largest endocrine organ in the body, producing myriad hormones and bioactive peptides. Signaling from the gut to the brain is carried out by highly chemosensitive neurons, immune cells, and specialized gut endocrine cells that produce over 30 hormones. Various classes of afferent neurons, for instance, exhibit receptors for hunger-generating (e.g., ghrelin) and satiety-generating (peptide YY, cholecystokinin, glucagon-like peptide 1, and oxyntomodulin) peptides that are secreted by enteroendocrine cells in the gut. According to animal studies, the expression of these receptors may be affected by nutritional status and diet. During periods of fasting, the expression of receptors for hunger-generating peptides is up-regulated, whereas the expression of receptors for satiety-generating peptides is down-regulated, demonstrating vagal afferent plasticity in response to a homeostatic state.

Chronic diseases, including inflammatory bowel disease and obesity, have been linked to dysregulation in gut-brain signaling. In obesity models induced by a high-fat diet, satiety-inducing gut-brain signaling mechanisms, such as the vagal afferent pathway, have been observed to be down-regulated. Imaging the brains of obese patients has revealed an increased sensitivity in neuronal pathways that predict reward in response to high caloric food cues and a decreased sensitivity to the actual effects/rewards of food intake in dopaminergenic pathways. This mismatch between expected and actual reward may describe a mechanism involved in food addiction and eating disorders. Another study found that the presence of intestinal microbiota influenced genes that regulate body fat in the hypothalamus and medulla, two brain regions that regulate body fat. The presence of body fat-inducing microbiota was also associated with symptoms of decreased hunger hormone leptin, which is produced by fat cells in proportion to fat mass to suppress appetite and may contribute to the relative obesity observed in conventional mice as compared to germ-free mice. In addition, the GI endocannabinoid system may play a role in regulating food intake. For instance, administration of a cannabinoid type 1 receptor (CB1) antagonist decreased food intake and weight gain in obese rodents, indicating that endocannabinoids may increase appetite. Consequently, the microbiota contributes to obesity by modulating gene expression and signaling in the central nervous system.

In addition to hormones, nutrients can communicate with the hypothalamus regarding food intake. Glucose and leucine, for instance, transmit satiety signals to the hypothalamus, whereas free fatty acids may induce satiety via ATP-sensitive potassium channels. Previously identified in the intestinal epithelium, guanylyl cyclase C receptors have been identified in the murine hypothalamus. Guanylyl cyclase C signaling is involved in gastrointestinal homeostatic mechanisms, such as anti-tumorigenesis, electrolyte balance, and barrier function. This aspect of the gut-brain endocrine axis may contribute to the association between obesity and colorectal cancer by regulating both energy balance and tumor suppression. Consequently, the brain, particularly the hypothalamus, plays a crucial role in appetite regulation, energy homeostasis, and the pathologies associated with obesity.

The gut microbiota, which is sometimes referred to as a forgotten organ, exists in high concentrations within the intestine, with approximately 1×10^{14} microbes residing in the colon. These organisms, both friend and foe, exist in close proximity to our immune system, of which approximately 80% resides in the gut. This high concentration of both microbes and immune cells requires highly complex interactions to maintain homeostasis. The gut microbes have key roles in the development of both the innate and adaptive arm of the immune system, gut motility regulation which determines rate of elimination, gut barrier function, fat deposit and distribution patterns and homeostasis.

Mind-altering microbes.

The following describes your brain on neurotransmitter-producing mood-altering microorganisms. The microbiota in the intestine can interact with chemical mediators, such as neurotransmitters like serotonin. Serotonin is produced in both neurons and the gastrointestinal tract. Previously, it was erroneously assumed that neurotransmitters only functioned within the central nervous system; however, we now understand that these signaling molecules have extensive and far-reaching effects at multiple sites. Neurotransmitters influence gut-related functions, including gut motility, nutrient assimilation, the innate immune system, and the gut microbiome. In addition to influencing mood, behavior, and cognition, the microbiota and neurotransmitters in the gastrointestinal tract also have a significant impact on other vital processes. In addition to producing a variety of neurotransmitters through the metabolism of plant fiber, gut bacteria also produce a number of neurotransmitters. *Bacillus* produces dopamine and noradrenalin, *Bifidobacteria* and *Lactobacilli* produce GABA, *Enterococcus* and *Streptococcus* produce serotonin, and *Escherichia* produces noradrenalin and serotonin.

The gut microbiota regulates a significant portion of the body's serotonin. Gut microbes alter neurotransmitter levels directly, which is one possible route of communication with neurons. It is intriguing that gut-derived metabolites stimulate serotonin production in the epithelial cells lining the large intestine, given that a number of antidepressant medications stimulate serotonin at neuronal junctions. Microbes in the intestine stimulate the biosynthesis of serotonin by specialized gut cells, which then supply serotonin to the intestinal epithelium and even platelets. Over 90 percent of human serotonin is produced in the gut. The hormone subsequently interacts with intestinal cells, enteric neurons, and immune cells.

The dysregulation of serotonin pathways can result in diseases such as irritable bowel syndrome and cardiovascular disease. On lymphocytes, monocytes, macrophages, and dendritic cells, serotonin receptors have been identified and are believed to play a role in immune signaling and modulation. The introduction of spore-forming microorganisms into the digestive tracts of germ-free rodents restores normal serotonin levels. When mice with natural microbiota were administered antibiotics, serotonin production decreased. Despite the fact that these are animal studies, they aid scientists in determining the cause-and-effect relationships. Uncertainty remains as to whether altered serotonin levels in the intestine influence brain activity. Intestinal inflammation or the development of gastrointestinal diseases such as Crohn's disease, ulcerative colitis, diverticulitis, and celiac disease may result from factors that inhibit serotonin expression.

Gut and blood barrier functions.

A healthy gut microbiota is necessary for the appropriate barrier function of the gastrointestinal mucosa and, consequently, for adequate immune defense. Numerous studies have demonstrated that colonization with or carriage of intestinal microbiota is essential for promoting normal immune responses. Germ-free mice lacking a gastrointestinal microbiota exhibited dysfunctional expression of certain toll-like receptors, which are responsible for detecting and distinguishing certain pathogenic bacteria from commensal species, and decreased IgA antibody secretion. However, when the intestinal mucosa was subsequently colonized in germ-free animals, the mucosal immune system was restored.

Recent neuroscience research has revealed that our microbiome regulates fundamental neurological processes. Microbes in the gut regulate the blood–brain barrier, neurogenesis, or the production of new brain cells, and the activation of microglia, which are immune cells in the brain and spinal cord. Previously, in science and medicine, it was believed that the brain was a privileged location that permitted only limited and restricted access. However, we now understand that intestinal microorganisms can communicate with the brain through both hard wiring and molecular signaling.

The physiology and permeability of the blood-brain barrier is influenced by metabolites derived from gastrointestinal microbes in rodents. Microbes in the gut break down fiber and carbohydrates into SCFA, which modulate the expression of tight junction proteins. For instance, the SCFA acid butyrate enhances the integrity of the blood–brain barrier by tightening the cell junctions. Thus, there is mounting evidence that both leaky gut and 'leaky brain' are influenced by the gut microbial community. In addition, gastrointestinal microbiota may influence the expression of brain-derived neurotrophic factor (BDNF), which is essential for the survival of extant neurons and the growth of new neurons, learning, memory, and higher cognitive processes. In animal models, the probiotic strains *Bifidobacterium breve* 6330 and *B. bifidum* breve 6330 as well as *B. longum* increased levels of BDNF. SCFA produced by microbes may influence BDNF expression and, by extension, numerous brain functions.

Bi-directional pathways of gut-brain regulation.

The gut microbiota may exert influence on the gut-brain axis via a number of bidirectional pathways. The gut-brain axis can be modulated by cortisol via the endocrine pathway, proinflammatory cytokines via the immune pathway, and the vagus nerve and enteric nervous system of the intestine via neural pathways. During periods of stress, the brain may also employ mechanisms within these pathways to regulate the composition of the gastrointestinal microbiome. The HPA axis of the brain regulates the release of cortisol, which can influence the immune system and inflammation, gastrointestinal permeability, and the community of the gut microbiota. The vagus nerve regulates numerous functions, including heart rate, aspects of respiration, and intestinal motility. Vagal nerve activation also produces an anti-inflammatory effect and has been demonstrated to be necessary for certain probiotics and endogenous intestinal microbes to exert health-promoting effects.

Numerous microbe-produced metabolites and microbe-derived components may influence gut-brain axis regulation. These microorganisms are able to produce modified bile acids, choline, and SCFA and regulate numerous aspects of our physiology. SCFA are neuroactive and stimulate the vagus nerve; they result from the microbial fermentation of complex carbohydrates. Probiotics, such as *Bifidobacterium infantis*, may modify the levels of kynurenine, which is an important component of the tryptophan (serotonin precursor) pathway in the context of oxidative stress. As previously mentioned, gut microorganisms can also produce neurotransmitters and neuromodulating compounds, including GABA, serotonin, dopamine, acetylcholine, and noradrenaline.

These microbe-produced neurotransmitters may then cause gut-lining epithelial cells to modify neural signaling or act directly on neurons. GABA is the primary inhibitory neurotransmitter in the brain, and its action on the vagus nerve may influence brain function. GABA reduces brain activity, and reduced levels are associated with anxiety and depression. *Lactobacillus rhamnosus* probiotic supplementation substantially increased GABA activity in the brain of rodents and altered their vagus nerve-dependent stress response. Additionally, microbes in the intestine regulate the expression and function of opioid and cannabinoid receptors in the gut. In patients with functional gastrointestinal disorders, the probiotic *Lactobacillus acidophilus* NCFM modulates mu-opioid receptor and cannabinoid receptor 2 (CB2) expression, reduces visceral pain perception, and reduces flatulence. The outer polysaccharide coating or cell wall carbohydrates of intestinal microorganisms are responsible for many of their health-promoting effects. The specialized cell wall of the probiotic strain *Bifidobacterium breve* UCC2003 protects it from the acid and bile in the gastrointestinal environment as well as the immune system.

Microbes and moods.

Many patients present with both gastrointestinal disorders and mood disorders at the same time, and the direction of causality has not been established. Despite decades of debate, the gut-brain axis is a bidirectional communication system. In fact, the relationship between gastrointestinal and mood disorders has been well-established for decades. Decades of population studies in IBS patients, for instance, have consistently reported high rates of psychiatric disorders; therefore, the presence of gastrointestinal symptoms is indicative of increased psychological distress. In addition, long-term investigations suggest that gut-brain connections are bidirectional. In a large study by Koloski et al., the presence of anxiety at baseline was predictive of a new gastrointestinal disorder at the 12-month follow-up among subjects without gut symptoms. At the 12-month follow-up, subjects with a gastrointestinal disorder but not a mood disorder at baseline had higher rates of anxiety and depression compared to controls. Moreover, in a 5-year database study conducted in the United Kingdom on patients who reported both a mood and gastrointestinal disorder, two-thirds of the subjects received a psychological diagnosis first, while one-third received a gastrointestinal diagnosis first.

Anxiety and depression increase sympathetic (fight-or-flight) and decrease parasympathetic (rest-and-digest) functions of the autonomic nervous system, which is crucial for the regulation of the enteric nervous system in the intestines. These conditions enhance the activity of the Hypothalamus-Pituitary-Adrenal (HPA) axis, leading to the upregulation of the stress markers cortisol and corticotrophin releasing factor. This results in a complex cascade of events, including increased inflammation and changes in the architecture of the gastrointestinal community and metabolic activity. Functional neuroimaging reveals that pain- and arousal-related brain regions are frequently aberrant in IBS patients. It has been shown that brain-focused treatments such as hypnosis and cognitive behavioral therapy reduce gut-related symptoms. Probiotics also exhibit therapeutic potential.

Stress negatively impacts gut microbes.

Stress modifies the activity of the autonomic nervous system, which in turn influences functions including gastrointestinal motility (transit time), inflammatory state, and immune function. In patients without physical disorder who have stress or depression, increased HPA axis activation, increased sympathetic with decreased parasympathetic tone, increased cortisol levels, and increased levels of inflammatory mediators disrupt homeostasis in the gut and microbiome. In disorders such as IBS, alterations in the intestinal microbiota may reflect a state of stress and heightened systemic inflammation. Neurotransmitters, such as norepinephrine (adrenaline), secreted in the gut in response to stress, increase the growth rate and modify the activity of a variety of disease-causing microbes. An increase in the population of pathogenic bacteria causes dysbiosis, which increases the risk of bacterial translocation across the intestinal lumen, leading to infections outside of the gut.

The notion that stress affects the gut microbiota and HPA axis has long been recognized and the specific functional effects of such changes are becoming clearer through ongoing basic research. Germ-free mice, which are

257

raised in sterile environments and therefore lack the normal endogenous microorganisms, exhibit an increased physiological response and reaction to stress compared to conventional mice harboring a microbiome. In addition, probiotic treatment could reverse the abnormal stress response in germ-free rodents. This was an early discovery that established the causal relationship between the microbiome and the optimal development of the HPA axis. In addition, the stress of maternal separation decreased the levels of beneficial intestinal *Lactobacilli* in Rhesus primates. Early-life stress can have significant and lasting effects on the microbiome, according to research. Both early life and chronic stress in adulthood are known to alter the composition of the gut microbiome and correlate with increased inflammation. Clearly, a healthy microbiome affects the development of an appropriate pattern of stress response later in life.

In addition to altering the composition and function of the gut microbiota, chronic stress impairs the integrity of the gut mucosal barrier, causing it to become permeable and allowing proinflammatory bacterial proteins to penetrate and gain access to the circulation. Probiotic treatment (such as *Lactobacillus* and *Bifidobacterium*) can reduce gastrointestinal permeability, abdominal pain, and inflammation, as well as stress-induced HPA axis dysfunction, according to accumulating research in rodents. In human investigations, intestinal permeability is linked to stress-related psychiatric disorders such as depression, highlighting the significance of the microbiota-gut-brain axis in regulating stress responses. In addition, specific species and strains of *Lactobacillus* and *Bifidobacterium* improve gut barrier function (i.e., diminish intestinal permeability) and rectify stress-induced changes to the HPA axis. A combination of *L. helveticus* R0052 and *B. longum* R0175 decreased cortisol levels in healthy humans. Treatment with prebiotics reduces the cortisol awakening response and emotional reactivity in healthy humans. It has also been demonstrated that *B. infantis* reduces stress-related behaviors in animals. This provides hope for the development of psychobiotics consisting of microorganisms and/or prebiotics to manage altered stress responses and enhance resilience.

Gut dysbiosis and bacterial infection of the intestine in a stressed patient may result in alterations in CNS function, behavior, and cognition, including learning and memory tasks. During and after eradication of infection, anxiety and cognitive impairment were observed in animal studies; these effects were prevented in probiotic-treated animals. In patients with irritable bowel syndrome (IBS), bacterial dysbiosis and stress appear to have a synergistic effect on gut-brain signaling and cognitive functions. In addition, accumulating evidence suggests a link between altered stress responses, alterations in immune regulation, and the prevalence of symptoms in IBS patients. Animal models have implicated the vagus nerve in gut-brain signaling during infections with a variety of opportunistic organisms. In instances where clinical validation is required, care must be taken not to extrapolate findings from animals to humans or from one bacterial strain to another.

The various pathways (e.g., vagus nerve dependent or independent) by which particular infectious organisms signal the brain are still being elucidated in greater detail.

Our cognition is influenced by microorganisms, and even the development of cognition is dependent on microbes. Studies on animals have demonstrated that the presence of microorganisms is necessary for the maturation of brain regions associated with memory. The probiotic *Bifidobacterium breve* NCIMB702258 increased the levels of the important for memory and learning fatty acids arachidonic acid (AA) and docosahexaenoic acid (DHA) in the brain. In addition, it has been observed that the geriatric and patients with cognitive disorders have a low diversity of species and ecosystem complexity in their digestive tracts.

Our gut microbiota may influence our behavior, brain chemistry, mood, and susceptibility to stress-related disorders like depression and anxiety. Clinical evidence supports the use of probiotics to enhance mood and reduce stress in healthy individuals, as well as improve stress responses in patients with chronic fatigue and irritable bowel syndrome. In healthy humans, supplementation with *Bifidobacterium* and *Lactobacillus* (such as *L. helveticus* and *B. longum*) reduces anxiety, depression, and stress-related behaviors. This probiotic supplementation was associated with decreased cortisol, anxiety, and depression levels, even in humans with minimal stress levels. Consuming fermented dairy products has also been associated with healthy brain function in humans.

The supplementation of diet with probiotics increases the levels of fatty acids in the brain, which are essential for brain function, learning, memory, and neurogenesis, or the creation of new brain cells. One multi-strain probiotic (i.e., *Bifidobacterium lactis*, *Lactobacillus bulgaricus*, *Streptococcus thermophilus*, and *Lactobacillus lactis*) was found to alter brain activity in the insula, an area involved in the regulation of mood in humans. Data in both animals and humans suggest that probiotics, often through a strain-specific effect, can therapeutically modulate brain function and behavior via the various communication routes of the microbiota-gut-brain axis.

Recent research on academic stress used *L. casei* Shirota treatment in which healthy students were given probiotics or a placebo for two months prior to medical school exams. The day before the examination, the probiotic-treated group had significantly lower cortisol levels than the placebo group. In addition, the probiotic group had significantly higher serotonin levels in the intestines two weeks after the exam. Another clinical trial on student athletes treated with *L. gasseri* OLL2809 LG2809 reported increased positive mood and reduced natural killer cell activity compared to the placebo group after strenuous exercise.

The psychological state of a patient, such as stress level, as a major determinant of treatment response has not been given full consideration in the context of conventional medicine. Scientists have discovered why chronic stress exacerbates gut symptoms in chronic conditions like inflammatory bowel disease (IBD) to increase abdominal pain, diarrhea, and fatigue. Brain-produced chemical signals released in response to chronic stress initiate a cascade of events that ultimately activate a large number of immune cells in the intestines. These cells secrete molecules that would ordinarily combat pathogens but instead cause excruciating bowel inflammation. The brain-gut-immune communication along the gut-brain axis in the context of chronic stress necessitates further investigation to fully elucidate this connection and its impacts on disease. The emergence of an evidence-based foundation for the mind-body connection should motivate both health care providers and funding agencies to understand more in the context of these conditions.

Microbes and pain.

In addition to behavioral disorders and cognitive impairment, the gut microbiota and gut-brain signaling are relevant in the context of other disorders such as pain. Specifically visceral or abdominal pain is often pronounced and debilitating in gastrointestinal disease such as IBS. Visceral pain and the perception thereof are complex. Interestingly, several brain areas process both visceral pain and psychological stress. In IBS patients, neuroimaging studies have revealed that brain regions such as the prefrontal cortex, a key area for abstract thought and behavioral regulation, are important in the pathophysiology of IBS. Some IBS patients also have altered brain activation during gut distention and altered expectations of discomfort. These patients have increased brain activation in regions that process information coming from the organs, increased emotional arousal, and altered inhibitory modulation of the experience and reactivity to pain. Additional studies are needed to understand whether the changes in brain structure and function in IBS are a consequence of increased gut-brain signaling or whether they have a causal role in pain amplification and deregulated gut function.

Ongoing research suggests that the gut microbiota affects the perception of abdominal pain. Many different probiotics, including those species from *Lactobacillus* and *Bifidobacterium*, have been shown to reduce abdominal pain in healthy humans and those with IBS. Animal studies have shown that probiotics such as *B. infantis* 35624 and *L. acidophilus* reduce visceral pain thresholds. In addition, animal studies reveal potential neural mechanisms of pain regulation. For example, *Lactobacillus* species have been shown to confer increased neuronal excitability in the gut and gut motility. In a human clinical trial, subjects with an abnormal ratio of interleukin-10 to interleukin-12, which indicates a heightened pro-inflammatory state, were treated with *B. infantis* 35624, *L. salivarius* UCC4331, or placebo. Only the *B. infantis* 35624 probiotic-treated group gained a normal inflammatory ratio post-treatment compared to the placebo group. These results indicate both that probiotics elicit changes in inflammation status in humans and such effects may be specific to particular groups or strains of microbes. However, no clear evidence exists to suggest which or why one probiotic group would be more beneficial compared to another for this purpose. Additional studies are required to elucidate relevant neural mechanisms and gut microbiota effects on brain function and pain.

Microbes and eating disorders.

In the industrialized world, eating disorders and the deregulation of eating behavior are prevalent. Those with anorexia nervosa are preoccupied with food but refuse to consume it, in contrast to those with obesity who ingest beyond their caloric requirements due to cravings. Numerous factors contribute to the pathology of obesity, including the central regulation of food intake (homeostasis versus hedonism), diminished cortical inhibitory mechanisms, and gut-based peripheral regulation. In addition to insulin and leptin (satiety hormone) resistance and altered vagal activation during food ingestion, an obese diet may elicit a reduction in gut-to-brain signaling that promotes satiety. Neuroimaging studies of obese patients reveal increased sensitivity in reward pathways in the brain in response to food cues such as seeing rich or preferred foods that predict reward but decreased sensitivity and decreased actual reward in dopamine pathways as a result of consuming the food.

Diet may play a role in the neurological changes that lead to these alterations in reward pathway regulation and decreased gut-to-brain signaling. Brain and behavioral abnormalities have been reported in patients with

265

anorexia. Subjects with anorexia nervosa have decreased activity in brain regions responsible for homeostatic activity and gut-to-brain signaling in response to feeding, but there is no correlation between this activity and perceived reward. This suggests that changes have occurred in which gut-to-brain signaling has a diminished effect on these patients' behavior and its modification. More research is required to comprehend changes in gut-brain and vagal signaling in this population. Neurological alterations may result in a disparity between the anticipated reward and the actual reward in obesity and food addiction. This disparity between anticipated and actual reward may lead to excess in an attempt to attain the expected reward level.

Microbes and autism.

Children with autism spectrum disorders (ASD), a neurodevelopmental disorder that may be linked to gut dysbiosis, frequently exhibit gastrointestinal symptoms. Some patients with autism spectrum disorder have altered gastrointestinal microbiota composition and short chain fatty acid levels, which are metabolic products of neuroactive bacteria. In animal models, probiotic treatment with *Bacteroides fragilis* and *Lactobacillus reuteri* can restore gut microbiota health. In animal studies, administration of the SCFA butyrate reduced repetitive behaviors, whereas administration of the SCFA propionate increased such symptoms.

According to studies, the elimination of gluten and casein from the diet reduces ASD symptoms.

Recent research has focused on investigating the effects of promising probiotic strains in individuals with autism. Certain strains of *Bifidobacterium*, such as *B. breve* and *B. longum*, have demonstrated potential benefits in improving gastrointestinal symptoms, reducing inflammation, and alleviating behavioral issues in children with autism. Similarly, various *Lactobacillus* strains, including *L. acidophilus* and *L. plantarum*, have shown promise in improving gastrointestinal symptoms, behavior, and cognitive function in individuals with ASD. *Streptococcus thermophilus* has exhibited potential immunomodulatory effects, improving gastrointestinal symptoms and behavior in individuals with autism.

Although research in this area is still emerging, several clinical studies and case reports have shown promising results. Probiotic interventions have been associated with improvements in gastrointestinal symptoms, social interactions, communication, and behavioral issues in some individuals with autism. However, further research is needed to better understand the role of microbiota and refine probiotic interventions for autism.

The era of psychobiotics.

The development of psychobiotics for the enhancement of mood and stress-related symptoms is a promising area of translational research. Psychobiotics are probiotics and/or prebiotics that alter the composition and/or activity of the gastrointestinal microbiota and provide the patient with a mental benefit. Psychobiotic treatment does not have to be limited to clinical populations with a diagnosed mental health disorder; it can also be used to enhance mental health indicators such as mood in healthy individuals, based on research conducted on healthy humans. As prebiotics can alter the composition and function of endogenous gut microorganisms, they hold promise as both co-administered and stand-alone interventions.

Psychobiotics exert their effects through various mechanisms that impact anxiety and other mental health symptoms. Probiotics can produce neurotransmitters, such as gamma-aminobutyric acid (GABA), serotonin, and dopamine, which are involved in mood regulation. Modulating these neurotransmitters may contribute to anxiety reduction. Probiotics can mitigate inflammation in the gut and throughout the body, as systemic inflammation has been linked to anxiety and other mental health disorders. Probiotics can strengthen the gut barrier, preventing the translocation of harmful substances into the bloodstream and reducing the release of pro-inflammatory molecules that may influence anxiety and other mental health symptoms.

Recent human trials of psychobiotics have focused on enhancing cognitive processes, HPA axis regulation, inflammation, and neural effects based on neurotransmitters (such as GABA and glutamate) and proteins (such as BDNF or brain-derived neurotrophic factor). A 30-day randomized controlled trial of a two-strain probiotic containing *Lactobacillus helveticus* R0052 and *Bifidobacterium longum* reduced cortisol levels, negative mood, and tension in healthy human subjects. Another recent clinical trial using a probiotic containing multiple strains of *B. bifidum* W23, *B. lactis* W52, *L. acidophilus* W37, *L. brevis* W63, *L. casei* W56, *L. salivarius* W24, and *L. lactis* W19 and W58 for 30 days reported decreased reactivity to negative mood, which was associated with decreased rumination and aggressive cognition, compared to the placebo group.

Specific strains have shown promise in targeting anxiety symptoms. *Lactobacillus rhamnosus* has been associated with reductions in anxiety-like behaviors and improved stress responses in preclinical studies, suggesting its potential as an anxiety-alleviating probiotic. For example, LGG is one of the most extensively studied probiotic strains and has been associated with various health benefits. While the research on LGG specifically targeting anxiety is limited, studies have shown its potential to modulate the gut-brain axis and improve stress responses, which may indirectly impact anxiety symptoms. *Lactobacillus rhamnosus* R0011 has been investigated for its potential effects on stress, mood, and anxiety-related behaviors. Studies suggest that *L. rhamnosus* R0011 may modulate stress responses and improve cognitive performance. However, more research is needed to determine its specific effects on anxiety.

Research suggests that *Bifidobacterium longum* may have anxiolytic effects by modulating the gut microbiota and influencing neurotransmitter production, promoting a calm and balanced mood. *Bifidobacterium longum* NCC3001 has been studied for its potential effects on stress-related behaviors and anxiety. Research suggests that *B. longum* NCC3001 may modulate the gut-brain axis, reduce stress-induced responses, and improve anxiety-related behaviors in animal models. However, further research is needed to determine its efficacy and safety in humans. In addition, *Bifidobacterium longum* 1714 has been investigated for its potential effects on mood and psychological well-being. Clinical trials suggest that *B. longum* 1714 may have anxiolytic properties, potentially reducing anxiety-related symptoms. Clinical studies have also indicated that *Lactobacillus plantarum* strain PS128 may alleviate anxiety by regulating the HPA axis, which plays a key role in the body's stress response. While these strains show great promise, more rigorous clinical trials are necessary to establish their precise effects on anxiety and determine optimal recommendations for their use.

Recent meta-analyses have demonstrated the potential for probiotic treatments to alleviate mild to moderate depressive symptoms in patients with multiple diseases. However, data on depressed patients remains scant. There is evidence that 90 days of *Bacillus coagulans* treatment improved depressive symptoms in patients with a dual diagnosis of major depressive disorder and irritable bowel syndrome. Clinical trials have reported that patients with major depressive disorder who took probiotics for 8 weeks reported a reduction in symptoms. Another recent meta-analysis indicated that probiotics are effective in reducing symptoms of depression when administered in combination with antidepressants but not when used alone.

Few studies have examined the effects of probiotics on the microbiota of the gut and cognitive functions in individuals with depressive symptoms, including IBS patients. Probiotic studies in IBS patients have reported an increase in the relative abundance of *Ruminococcus gauvreauii*, a decrease in the abundance of *Bacteroides* species, and an increase in microbial diversity in the gut. A randomized, controlled study published in Translational Psychiatry in 2022 found that consuming a high-dose probiotic containing eight distinct bacteria strains reduced depressive symptoms. However, it was emphasized that psychobiotics comparable to those used in the study should be considered in conjunction with therapy and not as a replacement for it.

Scientists are still attempting to determine the role of psychobiotics in the gut-brain axis and mental health, and more clinical studies are required to determine this role. A meta-analysis of 10 clinical trials involving probiotics and mental health was reported in 2020. All of the studies analyzed focused on individuals with stress, anxiety, or depression. While they found a positive correlation between probiotic use and a reduction in depressive symptoms, the correlation was not as robust when probiotics were used to treat anxiety. In addition, the probiotics had little effect on individuals experiencing acute stress in the trials analyzed. These contradictory results highlight the need to conduct further psychobiotic research.

Regarding pyschobiotics comprised of prebiotics in humans, one study used GOS (galactooligosaccharide), FOS (fructooligosaccharide), or a placebo to evaluate emotional appraisal and the psychophysiological effects of the prebiotics. Participants who consumed GOS exhibited a substantially enhanced cortisol awakening response, a biomarker for emotional disorders such as depression and stress. The GOS prebiotic also decreased vigilance, indicating a diminished response to negative emotions and potential antidepressant and antianxiety (anxiolytic) effects. These findings suggest that psychobiotics could be tailored to contain performance-enhancing properties as well as enhance mood and neural function.

While psychobiotics show potential for gut-brain axis disorders, it is important to adopt a holistic approach to mental health. Lifestyle modifications, including a balanced diet with adequate fiber and plants, regular exercise, stress management techniques, and professional guidance, should be considered alongside probiotic interventions. Moreover, additional research is necessary to fully elucidate optimal probiotic formulations, dosages, and their potential synergistic effects with existing treatments.

Microbial metabolites.

While the pathways of the microbiota-gut-brain axis are still being fully elucidated, evidence suggests that bacterial cell wall sugars, bacterially produces metabolites such as short chain fatty acids and neurotransmitters, vagal activation, and microbial modulation of the immune system are involved. Both direct physical interactions between gut microbes and the host as well as microbial metabolites exert potent effects. Short chain fatty acids, for instance, influence gastrointestinal processes such as gut motility, immune system development, and hormonal secretion. Some *Lactobacillus* species produce nitric oxide, which regulates the immune and nervous systems, whereas others produce neurotransmitters such as GABA. To determine the effects of various probiotic strains on the gut-brain axis, additional research is necessary. Understanding the communication mechanisms of the microbiota-gut-brain axis will accelerate the development of microbial therapeutics for the CNS and psychobiotics for mood disorders.

Therapeutic modulation of the gut-brain axis.

Animal and human studies using prebiotics and probiotics have demonstrated that psychobiotics can reduce psychiatric symptoms such as depression and anxiety. Even short-term changes in dietary patterns may induce rapid and large changes in the composition of the microbiome, which is relevant in these conditions. The development of probiotics and psychobiotics has been expanded to include potential treatment of gastrointestinal disease, obesity and other eating disorders, cognitive impairment and age-related decline.

The clinical research on psychobiotics highlights their potential as a novel approach to addressing mental health conditions. Promising findings indicate that specific probiotic strains may offer benefits in depression, anxiety, stress management, and cognitive function. However, further research is needed to establish evidence-based guidelines, optimize strain selection and dosages, and understand the underlying mechanisms. With continued exploration and rigorous clinical studies, psychobiotics may revolutionize mental health care by harnessing the power of the gut-brain connection.

The gut microbiome is extremely sensitive to diet and exercise, and since both affect mood, cognitive processes, and vagus nerve activity, the latter should also be explored for its pyschobiotic effects in human subjects. In Chapter 17, some Ayurvedic strategies for a healthy vagal tone are presented. While the field of psychobiotics is exciting and shows great promise for the treatment of psychiatric illness, cognitive decline, as well as the improvement of mood in healthy people, further studies are needed to fully translate the findings into clinical treatments. However, while some technical and translational limitations must be overcome, the current mechanistic insights show promise for the emergence of highly efficacious psychobiotics and the targeted, therapeutic modulation of the gut-brain-microbiome axis in the near future.

Part 3
Empowering Health through Microbial Change

You are what you both digest and absorb.

Chapter 12
Nutraceuticals: Wonder Drugs or Snake Oil?

Identifying health-promoting compounds present in natural sources, isolating those compounds in purified form, and packaging them as commercial supplements is becoming increasingly popular. The term nutraceutical combines nutrition and pharmaceutical. A nutraceutical is a pill, powder, or liquid that is ingested to promote health or treat disease. The premise underlying the health benefit of nutraceuticals is that they supply compounds in concentrations that would be challenging to obtain through the consumption of normal portions of fresh fruits and vegetables.

The widespread allure of nutraceuticals stems from the fact that they are derived from natural botanical sources, thereby decreasing the likelihood of adverse side effects associated with pharmaceutical medications. Examples of nutraceuticals include: vitamins, minerals, phenols such as resveratrol, and coumarins. Nutraceuticals also consist of complex mixtures derived from whole plants and fruits such as cranberry extract, the Ayurvedic herb Ashwagandha, and numerous others. Rapid growth is observed in the demand for these products, which are primarily derived from botanicals. By 2027, the global market for nutraceuticals is anticipated to surpass $261 billion.

The pertinent issue is whether or not nutraceuticals provide the advertised health benefits to the growing number of consumers who use these products. There is no simple response to this important query. Thousands of nutraceuticals are currently on the market. Theoretically, the majority of nutraceuticals have the potential to promote health, but in practice, many factors can affect whether or not this is the case. We have just learned that single-molecule nutraceuticals may or may not promote health, depending on the microbiome of the patient. The ability of a drug or nutraceutical to be delivered in sufficient concentrations to their site(s) of action to achieve the desired physiologic change is the determining factor in its ability to positively affect health.

To obtain FDA approval, pharmaceutical companies are required to conduct extensive pharmacokinetic and pharmacodynamic analyses. Pharmacokinetics examines the impact of the organism (us and our microbiome) on the drug's metabolism, rate of absorption, dissemination, and clearance, whereas pharmacodynamics examines the impact of the drug on the target tissue(s) and pathways to determine the magnitude of the observed change. In essence, drug companies must demonstrate the efficacy of their products and, to the greatest extent possible, ensure minimal adverse effects. This type of rigor does not exist for nutraceuticals, and as a result, consumers place a greater amount of faith in the advertised health benefits.

You are what you both digest and absorb.

Some nutraceuticals fail to provide a health benefit, primarily as a result of inadequate assimilation. In many instances, the quantities of therapeutic compounds entering the bloodstream are insufficient to induce a significant biological change. Even the most potent botanical compounds are rendered virtually ineffective if they cannot be efficiently absorbed and reach physiologically significant concentrations in targeted human tissues. The maximum levels of absorption and assimilation are obtained by the formulation of quality products.

Some compounds, such as calcium, are known to be assimilated less efficiently as we age, but vitamin D can improve calcium absorption. Clearly, things can become quite convoluted. The lack of scientific data regarding the assimilation of many nutraceuticals or the required concentrations to obtain health benefits places the consumer in a precarious position. In addition, numerous nutraceuticals make rather vague health claims. In the absence of clinical trials approved by the FDA, companies are not permitted to make specific health claims. In the absence of such trials, many companies provide indirect evidence intended to make you believe the efficacy of their health benefits.

Show us the evidence.

Numerous unsuccessful attempts to cure disease have taught us that it is difficult to do so. Comparing the levels and activities of all the proteins and molecules present in a healthy cell and a tumor cell will undoubtedly reveal a comprehensive list of differences. The assumption that restoring one or more of the differences to those of a normal cell guarantees that the tumor cell will be transformed back into a normal cell is false; in fact, the probability that this will occur is vanishingly small.

Consumers must keep this in mind when contemplating the purchase of supplements that use this type of "evidence" to support health-related claims. The evidence, for example, that the consumption of a specific substance decreased the levels of a protein known to be dysregulated in diabetes should serve as a red flag. What is the significance of this change, and does it correspond to an improvement in glucose tolerance or insulin sensitivity? If such information does not exist, a connection may not exist.

The preceding discussion is not meant to imply that all nutraceuticals are ineffective and provide no health benefits. In fact, many of them may offer substantial health benefits. Why, then, is it so difficult to distinguish between beneficial natural medicines and snake oil? The primary difficulty lies in the fact that, over the past several decades, scientific explorations have been skewed toward the study of disease, not health. This is not a criticism of our scientific priorities, but it has resulted in a disparity between our relative level of sophistication in comprehending the critical parameters that cause disease compared to those that keep us healthy.

The abundance of disease-related data and knowledge has provided the foundation for diagnostic innovations that permit rapid disease characterization and subclassification. They provide a logical method for developing more effective therapeutic intervention strategies to treat disease. The discovery of dysregulated pathways facilitates the discovery of new drug targets. To remedy the dysregulated pathway, pharmaceutical companies then seek to develop drugs that selectively stimulate or inhibit affected targets.

The quest for perfect health.

Since the financial implications are so high, the traditional drug discovery process is logical and rational despite its high rate of failure. Simply put, the foundation for uncovering therapies to improve the health of a clinically healthy person is not nearly as robust as our understanding of how to improve the health of the sick. The reasons are straightforward. The funders of scientific research have limited resources and are more inclined to give $1 million to a brilliant scientist with novel ideas for curing a disease than to the same scientist with equally excellent ideas for improving or maintaining the health of the healthy. It is difficult to refute that reasoning.

Many healthy individuals are aware that being regarded healthy by a physician simply means that measured health parameters lie within what is considered the normal range. Health has also been defined as merely the absence of disease and in populations that may not be optimally healthy. While normality is excellent news, for some individuals it is not enough; they strive to be greater than normal for optimal health and well-being.

Diet and exercise are significant strides in the correct direction toward optimal health, but what other reasonable options exist to achieve this objective? Sleeping well, stress management, and maintaining a positive emotional and mental state are also significant areas of focus that will likely pay off. But can optimal health be achieved with a pill, tonic, or cream? Perhaps, but these options are considerably less reliable, and scientific evidence is generally insufficient to make any choice certain.

It is impractical and probably irresponsible to make unequivocal judgements of the myriad health products available today. Products that work well for one individual may have little or no benefit to another. A smart consumer does their homework with an eye toward critical thinking. What is the evidence that a supplement will help? Is it limited to evidence derived from cells grown in a culture dish? Or are their animal and human studies that provide more direct evidence for their use and benefits? Ultimately, the individual consumer must play the role of judge and may require systematic testing of products that let you know whether your symptoms are alleviated or not. Avoid the mistake of trying multiple solutions at the same time. If you benefit from these interventions, you won't easily be able to know which supplement to attribute your improved health to. Patience and systematic explorations are the ley to finding products that work for you.

In the last section of the book, we examine in detail a number of powerful options for gut health. Perhaps some of the earliest medical practices viewed disease as something to be prevented. In the West, this particular perspective is uncommon, and corporations have little incentive to develop effective preventative therapies. There simply is not the same magnitude of return on investment. For those interested in being as healthy as possible it is worthwhile to explore the world of herbs.

Ayurveda and traditional Chinese herbal medicine were founded on the principle of targeting systems that can become subtly unbalanced in a global manner. Once systems become imbalanced, disease may begin to manifest. There is a strong inherent notion underlying these practices that if your systems are in a state of homeostasis, disease cannot manifest. This is a bold belief but nevertheless is not contradicted by what we know about chronic disease driven by environmental factors.

Chronic constipation is a serious medical issue that should not be disregarded or dismissed as a mere inconvenience.

Chapter 13
Changing your Microbiome with Probiotics: Probiotics to Maintain Human Health and Reverse Disease.

In ancient cultures, the consumption of fermented foods has been documented. These foods were undoubtedly preferred due to their resistance to spoilage. The process by which the naturally occurring microorganisms on these substances begin to break down the sugars in food or milk is called fermentation. This process acidifies the food, making it difficult for less acid-tolerant microbes that cause spoilage to thrive. According to records dating back 10,000 years, virtually all ancient civilizations consumed fermented milk products. Beyond the practical aspect of food preservation, cultures began to acknowledge the health benefits of fermented foods. Hippocrates, a Greek physician who lived from 460 to 370 B.C. and reached the age of 90, believed that fermented milk products were therapeutic. The Roman naturalist Plinius proposed using fermented milk products to treat gastroenteritis in the first century A.D. Fermented foods gained popularity because, in many cases, they acquired a pleasant flavor and texture and frequently became a part of the cuisine of the local culture. It is fascinating to consider that the very same bacteria that were responsible for fermenting these foods are now sold as probiotics in health food stores.

In 1680, the Dutchman Antonie van Leeuwenhoek was the first to observe yeast cells developing in fermenting beer, although no formal connection was made between the yeast's activities and the production of alcohol. A century passed before Lavoisier, a French chemist, figured out the process of sucrose metabolism and how it generated acids, ethanol, and carbon dioxide, but he did not realize that yeast cells were carrying out this complex chemistry. Louis Pasteur did not realize that fermentation could only occur in the presence of microscopic organisms until the late 1850s. The Russian scientist Ilya Ilyich Metchnikoff formalized the science of fermented foods at the turn of the 20th century. The foundation of his work was the observation of the excellent health and longevity of Bulgarian peasants who ingested copious amounts of yogurt rich in *Lactobacillus*, a common probiotic bacterium of the modern era. Metchnikoff's findings were published in a paper titled "The Prolongation of Life" Metchnikoff is widely regarded as the progenitor of modern probiotics, as a significant portion of his Nobel Prize-winning research involved elucidating the effect of ingesting live bacteria on the human immune system.

In addition to fermented substances, probiotics have entered the modern lexicon. A probiotic is a live microorganism that, when consumed, confers health benefits on the host. Many available probiotics contain numerous species of bacteria, primarily Lactic Acid Bacteria (LAB), *Lactobacillus*, and *Bifidobacterium*, as well as *Streptococcus* and other species. The use of these commercial products or specific strains of microorganisms has been analyzed in reasonable depth. Large meta-analyses (The analysis of datasets generated by multiple independent studies as an aggregate objective evaluation of the efficacy of a conclusion) of various probiotic species involving large numbers of human volunteers occasionally reveal disagreement in the conclusions reached by separate studies.

Several probiotics have a significant and reproducible positive effect on various aspects of human physiology.

Some species of *Bifidobacterium* impart increased resistance to bacterial infections and a reduction in diarrheal symptoms following the administration of antibiotics. Other strains of *Bifidobacterium* have the potential to enhance a number of immune system characteristics and promote anti-inflammatory signals that reduce systemic inflammation. Multiple studies support the immune modulatory potential of *Bifidobacterium* species, indicating a degree of heterogeneity in the therapeutic efficacy of probiotics across studies. Despite belonging to the same species, differences in the specific strains used are likely to account for the majority of this heterogeneity. Let's understand what strain variation means.

What's a probiotic?

Bifidobacterium longum is a prevalent probiotic species. In this instance, *Bifidobacterium* is the genus that contains over 30 recognized species, one of which is *B. longum*. Further, all bacterial species can be subdivided into strains that have undergone independent evolution, which typically involves the acquisition or loss of genes that distinguish it from its ancestors. Studies examining the number of strains belonging to a species of interest have reached a startling conclusion: the number of strains that have evolved is exceedingly large. A comparison of the complete genome sequences of two randomly chosen *B. longum* genomes reveals that strains belonging to the same species encode a remarkably high proportion of unique genes, typically 20-30% of the total number of genes. Adding a third, fourth, and so on to the comparison has no effect on these tendencies, as the total number of unique genes increases rather linearly.

The picture that emerges is a new appreciation of the large genetic heterogeneity of bacterial strains and the massive gene pools encoded by the species. This understanding has important implications for the consumer of probiotics as it is important to pay close attention to the specific strain of e.g., *Bifidobacterium longum* strain HF51, where HF51 is the strain designation. The health benefits of strain HF51 do not necessarily hold true for another *B. longum* strain KL88. While the basic properties of *Bifidobacterium* strains should be similar, they often differ in important features that determine their impact on human physiology. Some of the variable qualities are of practical importance like growth in large-scale industrial fermentation and survival post-production and upon consumption as it faces the strong challenges of passage through the hostile stomach and small intestinal environment. In the end, the efficacy of a strain depends on its ability to maintain sufficient survival and to modify the intended immune and biochemical pathways of the host in order to positively impact human health.

The variability of probiotic strains is the primary reason for the lack of consensus regarding their therapeutic value. Commercial producers of probiotics are in the business of making a profit, and as a result, they look to market the strains they have acquired and characterized. Some strains exhibit efficacy when objectively evaluated by independent scientists, while others do not. Since relatively few studies explicitly compare one strain to another and compare multiple strains, it is difficult to completely comprehend the mixed results of such evaluations. Similarly perplexing is the fact that each investigation of probiotics employs various models of efficacy, some using cell-based models, others using rodent models, and still others employing human trials. In addition, the endpoints of these studies frequently vary, making it nearly impossible to distinguish between strains with genuine health benefits and those without. The best studies are those that measure the objective and direct impact of disease prevention on human volunteers. Human cell culture studies, while useful to the scientist as a step toward a greater understanding of the mechanisms by which probiotics may achieve therapeutic effects, are not particularly informative to the consumer, as they do not provide any evidence that the probiotic has the ability to maintain health or reverse complex disease.

While the probiotic industry has grown rapidly over the past several years, clinicians have been slow to embrace probiotic therapies. There are valid reasons for this, as the efficacy of individual strains to treat specific and well-defined human conditions varies greatly. The increasing prevalence of probiotics may be indicative of the growing number of individuals who recognize that their digestive health is not optimal. One ability generally attributed to the majority of probiotics is the restoration of intestinal health. Despite the fact that this is a relatively imprecise health claim, probiotic companies are not permitted to make more specific health claims without conducting multimillion-dollar clinical trials to support those claims. The purpose of these regulations is to protect consumers from false health claims. This is in everyone's best interest, but it has the unfortunate side effect of delaying the aggressive development of probiotics capable of treating specific disease conditions. There is little or insufficient incentive for companies to conduct expensive clinical trials with their products in order to make a definitive statement about the clinical impact of their product. This unfortunately makes it difficult for consumers to acquire the best products and avoid the worst.

There are specific aspects of gastrointestinal health that are supported by robust scientific evidence. The majority of independent studies evaluating the efficacy of probiotics concur that probiotics have a positive effect and are recommended after an oral antibiotic course. Antibiotics are used to eliminate bacterial pathogens. For years, this was the extent of our understanding, but we now know that antibiotics also destroy a significant portion of the intestinal microbiota. One of the functions ascribed to the gut microbiota is the process of pathogen exclusion, wherein resident commensal microbes occupy sites that pathogenic bacteria need for infection. When the microbiota is eradicated by antibiotics, the intestine becomes susceptible to secondary infections, particularly those caused by infectious agents that are drug-resistant. Probiotics have shown efficacy in protecting individuals from pathogens after antibiotic use, and they also mitigate diarrhea, which frequently follows antibiotic use.

Understanding the effects of constipation.

Human trials that required participants to provide a daily stool sample, revealed that numerous stools were firm and severely dehydrated, indicating excessive stool retention and constipation. The severity of constipation varies, and those suffering from severe constipation experience discomfort, bloating, and lethargy, negatively affecting their quality of life. Constipation increases the risk of developing more serious diseases, such as colorectal malignancies, in addition to the discomfort it causes.

Historically, it was understood that stool retention promoted a process known as putrefaction. Today, we recognize this process as something that occurs in individuals with excessive stool transit times, in which anaerobic fermentation of protein extends beyond what is normal, resulting in the production of compounds with a noxious odor, which is an additional complication of constipation. Unfortunately, some of these products are mutagenic and, if generated in sufficient concentration, can cause mutations in colonic cells and their stem cells, the progenitors of all colonocytes. Other mutations are so detrimental to cellular function that they induce programmed cell death, thereby preventing the harmful mutation from spreading as cells divide. A small percentage of mutations may modify oncogenes or tumor-suppressor genes, which, when functionally disrupted, predispose individuals to tumor development. In this regard, chronic constipation is a serious medical issue that should not be disregarded or dismissed as a mere inconvenience. Numerous independent studies have demonstrated that probiotics are useful for relieving constipation.

Probiotics for health and disease.

Several additional conditions, including atopic disease, irritable bowel syndrome, and others, show promise and potential for probiotics to alleviate disease symptoms. Probiotics have the potential to reduce the growth rate of tumors in animal models of melanoma and hepatocellular carcinoma (liver cancer) by a significant amount, according to several recent studies published in the most prestigious scientific journals. These unequivocal results appear to be at odds with probiotics' reputation as a weak therapeutic, which a rational person would compare to the finest pharmaceutical medications. In fact, one of these studies demonstrated that administering a *Bifidobacterium* species to rodents with melanoma tumors was as effective as a class of cancer immune-therapeutics in use today. Even more intriguing was the fact that the combination of probiotics and immune therapy had additive effects on tumor growth suppression. Are these results simply an aberration? How do we account for the differing perspectives regarding probiotics? What are we failing to consider?

Manufacturing challenges.

A closer examination of commercial probiotics provides a plausible, if not likely, explanation for why probiotics continue to be controversial and inadequately accepted by the medical community. The answers lay in the extraordinary difficulties associated with delivering a high dose of live bacteria to their site of action, which is typically the small intestine or colon. For the bulk production of probiotic bacteria, hundreds or thousands of liters of bacterial cultures are grown in fermenters to produce very large populations of bacteria. This process is stressful for the bacteria, which produce stress response proteins in order to defend themselves from the harm caused by high-density bacterial culture. These bacteria are harvested and dehydrated using patented methods. The bacteria are then packaged with great care to preserve their high viability prior to distribution. Labels for probiotics must indicate the number of viable microbes present in the product at the time of distribution. In general, the number of viable microbes per dose in the majority of probiotics is greater than 1×10^9. While the dose of a probiotic is essential to its ability to promote health, the number of live microbes at its site of action is of greater importance.

It is instructive to consider the probiotic's arduous voyage from the production facility to the consumer's colon in order to gain a better understanding of how long it takes for live bacteria in probiotics to reach their site of action after manufacture. *Bifidobacterium* and *Lactobacillus* are the most prevalent probiotic species used today, as we have learned. Their sensitivity to oxygen is a significant distinction between these bacterial strains. *Lactobacilli* are known as facultative anaerobes due to their ability to thrive in both aerobic (oxygen-containing) and anaerobic (oxygen-deficient) environments. *Bifidobacterium*, on the other hand, are strictly anaerobic bacteria that are extremely sensitive to even trace quantities of oxygen. This characteristic of *Bifidobacterium* poses a significant challenge for probiotic manufacturers who seek to minimize the loss of product viability by minimizing oxygen exposure throughout the manufacturing process.

To mitigate viability loss, probiotic manufacturers invest significant time and money in identifying probiotic strains that not only provide the desired health benefit, but also possess characteristics that improve viability retention during processing and shelf life after distribution. Various freeze-drying techniques are employed to maintain the utmost possible product viability; however, these obstacles are not the end of the tale. First, high-quality probiotics should be refrigerated to preserve their viability. In the event that this is not the case, there is a greater chance that the product will not have the desired effect.

The voyage of a probiotic through you.

Once consumed, microbes transition from a "suspended animation" state to a metabolically active cell. This transition is not uniformly efficient, and it is believed that this is due to the quantity and composition of stress proteins expressed by probiotic bacteria during the manufacturing process. Upon entering the stomach, these bacteria encounter a hostile environment, to say the least. The stomach's acidity can be as low as pH 1, but is typically between pH 2-3. While these distinctions may seem insignificant, it is crucial to remember that pH is measured on a base ten scale, meaning that there is 10 times more acid (H^+ ions) at pH 1 than at pH 2, and 100 times more acid at pH 1 than at pH 3. In addition to acid stress, the bacteria in probiotics encounter highly active enzymes in the stomach and small intestine that are designed to break down the food we consume into simpler substrates. In this assault, the bacteria in probiotics receive no quarter. It is unknown what proportion of probiotic bacteria survive passage through the stomach, but it is fair to presume that this harsh environment has the greatest impact on viability.

The survivors enter the small intestine, where they encounter additional obstacles in the form of digestive enzymes and bile acids produced by the liver and secreted by the small intestine. These bile acids have antimicrobial properties that may reduce the number of probiotic bacteria even further. The oxygen present in the stomach and small intestine is deleterious to *Bifidobacterium* probiotics and contributes to their loss of viability. Few studies have evaluated the viability of probiotics during transit through the gastrointestinal tract, but it is plausible that the loss of viability could be as high as 1×10^{-5} or more, which is equivalent to a loss of at least 99.99% of the initial dose. It is probable that probiotic bacteria's diminishing viability is directly related to their somewhat limited therapeutic potential. This is the same as any other drug. Would you anticipate to feel pain alleviation if you took 99.99% of the recommended dose of aspirin for a headache?

Our negative conclusions regarding the therapeutic potential of probiotics may be premature for these reasons. Despite the lengthy history of probiotics, we may not fully understand their ability to enhance human health and reverse disease. Future innovations and strategies may radically alter our perception of probiotics as the subsequent generation of pharmaceuticals. Below, we will discuss some of these ideas and characterize strategies that may enable consumers to derive greater benefits from existing probiotics and their own microbiome.

New probiotic developments.

New encapsulation technologies are being developed that may prevent loss of viability and permit the delivery of significantly higher concentrations of bacteria to their site of action. Encapsulation technologies involve coating desiccated probiotic preparations to protect them from oxygen, gastric acids, and digestive enzymes. As with time-release capsules, these encapsulated probiotics may remain intact until the probiotic reaches the small intestine or colon, depending on the condition being treated and where the bacteria's activity affects host physiology. Although numerous encapsulation technologies have been described in the scientific literature, they are not readily available in probiotic formulations. Encapsulation of probiotics may force consumers and health care providers to reconsider the use of probiotics to treat patients. Researchers continue to make thrilling new discoveries that expand the possibilities for bacterial-based therapeutics in our lifetime, so the list of diseases that may benefit from probiotics is not yet complete. In the future years, the essence of substances we currently refer to as drugs may undergo a significant transformation. Natural therapeutics, such as probiotics, are likely to be utilized more frequently as stand-alone treatments as well as adjunctive methods that are combined with conventional pharmaceutical medications.

An essential characteristic of probiotics is their transient therapeutic effect, as the bacteria ingested do not typically colonize the gastrointestinal tract permanently. When contemplating the use of probiotics for general digestive health versus chronic disease treatment, this fact must be taken into account. When using probiotics to treat short-term digestive issues such as diarrhea, constipation, or maintaining a healthy flora after antibiotic use, it makes perfect sense to choose a probiotic with solid double-blind human trials supporting its efficacy in treating your specific condition. Once the problem has been resolved, you can discontinue the probiotic and observe whether the symptoms return. If so, it is recommended that you consult your physician to discuss alternatives. The capacity of probiotics to produce cures (symptoms disappear and do not return) has not been adequately studied, and data on the frequency of recurrence or relapse are typically unavailable. If you intend to use probiotics on a long-term basis to maintain digestive health or as an adjunctive therapy to treat chronic disease, you must consider additional factors.

Probiotics are considered safe for long-term use, and adverse effects are rarely reported. For many, the modest daily expense (approximately $1 per day) of long-term probiotics to prevent gastrointestinal distress is justified by the benefits. It would be a shame if you weren't receiving the utmost benefit possible from your probiotic, despite the additional expense. It is essential to realize that a probiotic with demonstrated efficacy in reducing flatulence may be completely ineffective as a treatment for constipation, weight loss, or diabetes. It is prudent to identify the probiotic that is most suitable for the condition you desire to treat. Spend time conducting investigation. Avoid .com websites, as you can be certain that you are being targeted for marketing. Avoid probiotic literature that promotes probiotics, as the presentation may lack objectivity. If appropriate research has been conducted, you can be certain that scientists have compiled graphs, figures, and statistics based on their findings.

Probiotics and chronic diseases.

Autoimmune diseases such as psoriasis, rheumatoid arthritis, systemic lupus erythematosus, autoimmune thyroid disease, multiple sclerosis, immune thrombocytopenic purpura, vitiligo, and inflammatory bowel disease (IBD) are one area where probiotics show significant promise. Important immune cells known as regulatory T cells (Tregs) are diminished in these diseases. These cells serve a crucial role in maintaining immune homeostasis and preventing acute or chronic inflammation-induced tissue injury. In order to comprehend how these immune cells can be activated in the context of inflammatory diseases, a great deal of research has been conducted. Tregs produce cytokines that suppress inflammation. Intriguingly, Tregs are viewed as the adversary in the context of many types of solid tumor cancers, as their activity inhibits other immune cells from assaulting the tumor as they would normally. Gut organisms appear to intelligently communicate with the immune system, which may prevent this duality from causing damage to the host.

An integrative approach may include probiotics that have demonstrated clinical efficacy in IBS. *Lactobacillus plantarum* 299v improved global symptoms, abdominal pain and bloating in IBS patients. A probiotic barley extract with *Lactobacillus rhamnosus* NCIMB 30174, *L. plantarum* NCIMB 30173, L. acidophilus NCIMB 30175 and *Enterococcus faecium* NCIMB 30176 improved global symptoms in IBS subjects. In addition, *Streptococcus faecium* as well as a 4-strain probiotic containing *L. acidophilus* CUL60, *L. acidophilus*, *Bifidobacterium* animalis subsp. lactis CUL34 and *Bifidobacterium bifidum* CUL20 induced similar improvements in global symptoms. A 2-strain probiotic mix of *E. faecalis* DSM 16440 and *Escherichia coli* DSM 17252 improved global symptoms and abdominal pain in IBS patients. A 4-strain probiotic *Bifidobacterium animalis* subsp. *actis* BB-12®, *Lactobacillus acidophilus* LA-5®, *Lactobacillus delbrueckii* subsp. *bulgaricus* LBY-27 and *Streptococcus thermophilus* STY-31 improved global symptoms, abdominal pain and bloating. Another A 4-strain probiotic containing *Bifidobacterium bifidum* BGN4, *Bifidobacterium lactis* AD011, *Lactobacillus acidophilus* AD031 and *Lactobacillus casei* IBS041 as well as a 6-strain probiotic containing *Bifidobacterium longum*, *Bifidobacterium bifidum*, *Bifidobacterium lactis*, *Lactobacillus acidophilus*, *Lactobacillus rhamnosus* and *Streptococcus thermophilus* improved global symptoms and abdominal pain but not bloating in IBS. Current clinical recommendations for probiotics in IBS include that taking a probiotic product is considered safe in IBS and that probiotics are unlikely to provide substantial reduction in IBS symptoms. Additional clinical trials are needed to identify optimal probiotic treatment interventions and symptom reduction in IBS.

An integrative approach often includes probiotic treatment. Probiotics that have demonstrated clinical efficacy in reversing obesity include *Lactobacillus gasseri* SBT2055, *Lactobacillus* plantarum, yogurt containing *L. acidophilus* La5, *Bifidobacterium* lactis Bb12, and *L. casei* DN001. In obese women, a synbiotic (probiotic + prebiotic) containing *L. rhamnosus* CGMCC1.3724 with oligo-fructose and inulin supplementation promoted weight loss and reductions in circulating leptin, which is a hunger-promoting hormone. A combination of *bifidobacteria, Lactobacilli,* and *S. thermophilus* was shown to improve insulin sensitivity and lipid profiles in overweight subjects.

L. acidophilus La-5 and *B. animalis* subsp. *lactis* BB-12 administration was shown to decrease fasting blood glucose, cholesterol and LDL levels while increasing total antioxidant status in T2D patients. In a study on males with T2D, *L. acidophilus* NCFM improved insulin sensitivity. Clinical trials in T2D patients using bread containing a synbiotic of *L. sporogenes* and inulin reported decreased serum insulin and lipids with an increase HDL. A synbiotic shake containing *L. acidophilus, B. bifidum* and fructo-oligosaccharides was administered to elderly patients with T2D and led to reductions in fasting glycemia with increases in HDL. Many strains of probiotics show promise for the management and prevention of diabetes and obesity such as *Anaerobutyricum hallii*, *Akkermansia muciniphila*, and *Clostridium beijerinckii*.

Several investigations on the commensal bacteria *Bacteroides fragilis* in the intestine have demonstrated that this bacterium communicates with the immune system via outer membrane vesicles (OMVs). By compressing a small portion of the outer cell membrane, these vesicles are generated. These vesicles transport cargo, which may be laden with bioactive substances or convey whatever is present in the bacterial cytoplasm. The OMVs manufactured by *B. fragilis* possess a polysaccharide called polysaccharide A that influences the immune system in intriguing ways. Polysaccharide A induces Tregs in the local gut microbiome, indicating a beneficial function in suppressing inflammatory processes in the gastrointestinal tract. Interestingly, this molecule can induce T helper 1 (Th1) cells throughout the entire body. The Th1 cells may contribute significantly to stimulating the immune system's attack on tumor cells.

Presently, the FDA has not approved *B. fragilis* for use as a probiotic. Given the ability of this microorganism to preserve health and potentially alleviate disease, one is left to ponder whether it is possible to obtain *B. fragilis* despite the fact that this probiotic is not commercially available. It is likely that many other gut-dwelling bacterial species, such as various *Clostridia* and *Akkermansia* which have hit store shelves recently, possess a similar capacity to relay intricate instructions to the immune system or protect the gut. Recent studies have revealed many potential next generation probiotics. These include *Prevotella copri* and *Christensenella minuta,* which may regulate insulin resistance, *Parabacteroides goldsteinii, Bacteroides thetaiotaomicron,* and *Akkermansia muciniphila* which may reverse obesity and insulin resistance, *Faecalibacterium prausnitzii,* which protects mice from intestinal diseases, and *Bacteroides fragilis,* which reduces inflammation and exhibits anticancer properties. In the next chapter, which investigates the promise of prebiotics and their powerful effects on the gastrointestinal microbiome, these options will be discussed in greater detail.

For many years, commercially available probiotics were limited to bacteria belonging to just a few genera, e.g., *Lactobacillus* and *Bifidobacterium.* Intensive research of the gut microbiome focused on the role of individual species have led to the identification of numerous bacterial species displaying promise as next generation probiotics. In fact, some of these are starting to make their way onto the shelves of our favorite health food stores for purposes such as mental health and glucose control. Microbes with documented ability to reduce adiposity (fat), reduce inflammation (associated with most chronic diseases), improve cognitive function etc. are likely to be available to consumers in the coming years.

Perhaps the modulatory potential of polyphenolic compounds derives from their ability to alter host cell physiology, such as immune cell function, which in turn modifies the intestinal microbiota.

Chapter 14
Changing your Microbiome with Prebiotics

Prebiotics are an exciting domain that will likely gain popularity in the future years. A prebiotic is defined as a fiber that is not digestible by humans but modulates the gut microbiota and/or its activities in such a way as to confer a health benefit to the host. This definition has been slightly modified periodically and is a well-accepted definition. However, there are those who view the definition as overly restrictive as many natural compounds have gut microbiota modulatory capacity, making dietary fiber an extraneous component of the definition. Similarly, there are those who do not believe that prebiotics should be restricted to those for which the host has no capacity to metabolize. Both arguments have merit and will no doubt be discussed in future scientific congresses where it is likely the definition will undergo further revision. It seems the most important parts of the prebiotic definition are that it should be natural and have gut microbiota modulatory capacity that confers a health benefit to the host.

How do prebiotics work?

Polysaccharides are prebiotic carbohydrates that have a significant capacity to modulate the intestinal microbiota. Polysaccharides are composed of subunits of sugar. Some polysaccharides, such as starch, are basic glucose polymers, whereas others are more complex, containing a variety of sugars with a variety of chemical bonds. Gut microbiota metabolize both simple and complex polysaccharides in two distinct steps requiring the cooperation of multiple species. In order to be transported into bacterial cells, polysaccharides must first be broken down into oligosaccharides and monosaccharides. Multiple bacterial groups encode enzymes that decorate the cell surface. These enzymes recognize particular sugars and chemical bonds between sugars and catalyze the breakdown of long sugar polymers into simpler units, which can then be transported into bacterial cells and utilized as energy.

Some of the sugars liberated by bacteria can be directly metabolized by those same bacteria, while others cannot and serve as an energy source for other bacteria capable of transporting and metabolizing these additional sugars. In this regard, the complexity of carbohydrates in a prebiotic determines the diversity of bacterial species that stand to benefit from prebiotic ingestion. Inulin is by far the most extensively studied prebiotic fiber. Inulin is present in numerous plants, but chicory root is the primary commercial source. Inulin is a polymer of fructose with a glucose molecule at its terminal end. The observation that inulin consumption induces an increased abundance or "bloom" of *Bifidobacterium* spp., which are well-known components of many probiotics and considered beneficial, health-promoting bacteria, is one of the primary reasons for the biased study of inulin.

As sequencing technologies have advanced, it has become evident that inulin promotes the proliferation of additional bacterial species, such as *Bacteroides* and *Akkermansia* muciniphila. This is one of the principal benefits of prebiotics. They stimulate not only the growth and activity of probiotic species in the colon, but also the growth and activity of health-promoting species that are presently unavailable as probiotics due to FDA restrictions. The benefits of *A. muciniphila* for weight loss and appetite suppression have been discussed. Some Bacteroides species have considerable immune modulatory capacity, and *B. fragilis* has been shown to improve gut barrier function, thereby reversing leaky gut, a pathology that underlies a wide range of diseases for which there are presently no validated therapeutics.

In this regard, one of the most significant advantages of prebiotics is the utility of bacterial species that are unavailable as probiotics but appear to have significant potential to treat a wide range of diseases.

The specific species induced by inulin consumption are consistent with those bacteria encoding the necessary enzymes for their degradation, transport into the cell, and energy-producing metabolic pathways. Aside from a few additional dietary fibers such as starch, arabinoxylans, and a few others, the study of additional prebiotics is generally deficient in detail. Evident from these studies is that each prebiotic alters the gastrointestinal microbiota in a unique manner due to its unique sugar and chemical linkage properties. As we learn more about the health benefits of gut microbes, it becomes clear that prebiotics may be the key to modulating the composition of the gut microbiota in ways tailored to an individual's health requirements. The vast majority of complex carbohydrates found in common fruits, vegetables, and roots have not been studied for their modulatory effect on the gastrointestinal tract.

The prebiotics market.

It is puzzling, given the current efforts to expand the probiotic industry, that the study and commercialization of prebiotics have lagged so far behind. Unfortunately, the likely causes of this disparity are straightforward economics. It is challenging to obtain patent protection for naturally occurring plant compounds. Some manufacturers have developed patentable processes for generating prebiotics, but the inability to protect their product as firmly as a novel probiotic strain discourages biotechnology companies from pursuing this type of therapeutics. Hopefully, this trend will alter in the future, and both academic and commercial research will actively pursue the true potential of prebiotic compounds.

According to Chapter 12, polyphenolic compounds have been extensively examined for their health benefits. Given what we know about polysaccharide prebiotics, it is somewhat puzzling that a number of polyphenolic compounds appear to have intestinal microbiota modulatory capacity and, assuming they confer health benefits on the host, would satisfy the definition of a prebiotic substance. Since the consumption of polyphenolic compounds is not predicted to provide direct energy to bacterial cells, it is unknown how they modulate the intestinal microbiota. This raises the question of why bacterial species in the intestines possess and express enzymes with the specific function of transforming polyphenolic compounds into biochemical products with enhanced absorption and bioactivity. Perhaps the modulatory potential of polyphenolic compounds derives from their ability to

319

alter host cell physiology, such as immune cell function, which in turn modifies the intestinal microbiota. In this regard, prebiotics may be thought of as belonging to one of two classes, those that have direct effects on microbial fitness and those that have indirect effects.

Current and future studies on prebiotics.

To thoroughly characterize the gut modulatory capacity of a vast array of dietary compounds, much work remains. Everything we know about the effects of consuming fruits, vegetables, and the prebiotic components of these foods indicates that the positively affected microbes in the gut are species that have been implicated or directly shown to alter human physiology in a positive manner through increased SCFA levels, improved gut barrier function, and immune modulation, which may have a significant impact on a wide range of inflammatory diseases. This provides a substantial impetus for further scientific research and commercial production of prebiotic compounds.

One potential drawback of prebiotics is that their health benefits depend on the specific bacterial strains carried by each individual. To comprehend this, we refer to the voluminous research on the health benefits of probiotics. Numerous studies demonstrate that strains of bacteria belonging to the same species exhibit substantial variation. Comparing several strains of *Bifidobacterium longum* for their effects on immune stimulation, for instance, reveals that only a few strains have a significant effect on any metric of host physiology. This statement should be qualified, however, as any such comparison of strain efficacy is limited to the specific experimental evaluations conducted by the study in question. In other words, a *Bifidobacterium longum* strain that exhibited no positive effect on weight gain may have substantial potential to alleviate allergy or autoimmune disease symptoms. However, the health benefits of prebiotics experienced by an individual depend on the specific strains that an individual harbors.

By combining the appropriate prebiotic and probiotic, it is possible to combine the modulatory effects of prebiotics with the specific probiotic strains that have demonstrated health benefits. A synbiotic is a combination of prebiotics and probiotics. Despite the high perceived utility of this therapeutic approach, there are currently only a small number of studies on synbiotics. It is possible that synbiotics could provide a solution to the significant loss of bacterial viability that most probiotics experience during their passage through the stomach and small intestine. Once in the colon, synbiotics, if coupled with an appropriate prebiotic, could stimulate a significant proliferation of probiotic bacteria, combining the benefits of the prebiotic and the probiotic strains. The proliferation of probiotic bacteria in the colon occurs as a result of the so-called lunchbox effect, in which the bacteria are provided with an energy source tailored to their specific requirements.

The process of fermentation of dietary fibers generates H_2 and CO_2 gas. Some people who consume inulin experience discomfort and bloating due to excessive gas production. On the one hand, this symptom indicates that the prebiotic is doing its work, but those taking inulin for the alleviation of gastrointestinal discomfort may find this remedy counterproductive. The use of synbiotic formulations must be investigated in greater depth, as the possibility of even greater gas production exists if the proper bacteria are provided with a king's meal, which may result in the formation of extremely rapid fermentation products. Although these obstacles are not insurmountable, you should consult a physician before attempting this method. Some subjects have begun taking prebiotics at lower concentrations than recommended and have discovered that gradually increasing the dose over the course of two weeks alleviates sporadic bloating and discomfort.

Experimental evidence has been generated that highlights the power of prebiotics in a mouse melanoma model. Standard laboratory mice were provided prebiotics in their drinking water and subsequently injected with tumor cells subcutaneously. Mice not provided prebiotics developed large tumors over the course of 2-3 weeks, whereas the prebiotic fed mice developed tumors more slowly. When combined with antibodies used clinically to treat melanoma patients, the prebiotic treated mice displayed a synergistic activity stronger than either prebiotic alone or antibody treatment alone. Furthermore, these mice displayed a significant lag in the time it took for antibody treatment resistance to develop. Again, these results show the power of the microbiome via its response to prebiotics to have drug-like potency to treat disease.

In Chapter 15, we'll explore the powerful prebiotic effects of medicinal herbs. While the power of prebiotics to therapeutically modulate microbiomes is currently underappreciated, in the future, it remains likely that prebiotics could represent the preferred method to robustly increase healthy gut species and their activities in a sustainable manner.

Fortunately, there is no true separation of species, rather the interaction, collaboration and exchange of information and resources within an interconnected community.

Chapter 15
How Herbs Work: Changing Your Microbiome with Ayurvedic Herbs

Ayurveda is a term from the ancient Indian Sanskrit language meaning "knowledge of life' or "science of perfect health.' As the traditional Indian system of personalized medicine, Ayurvedic medicine prioritizes disease prevention, health promotion, and the reversal of disease. According to Ayurveda, diseases originate in the gastrointestinal tract. Through this lens, disease is identified at the earliest stage of pathogenesis, when imbalance first initiates and accumulates in the gut. This approach thus seeks to treat the root cause of disease in the digestive system early in the disease process.

Medicinal botanicals form the basis of an Ayurvedic treatment plan and are extensively prescribed in integrative medicine, but you may be wondering how they work. Herbs may promote therapeutic benefits through a variety of known and unknown mechanisms. The known mechanisms of action include the direct absorption of herb-derived molecules across the lining of our gastrointestinal tracts into the bloodstream, taste receptor signaling on both the tongue and intestinal walls, bacterial metabolism of herbs into bioactive constituents, and the secretion of additional health-promoting substances, known as post-biotics, molecules produced by the microbes as the result of metabolizing the herbs.

Herbs are polymolecular medicines

We must keep in mind that medicinal herbs are plants with complex profiles that produce polymolecular medicines with far-reaching effects on multiple targets and body systems, as opposed to single-drug or single-nutraceutical approaches that affect single targets. Many of the botanicals commonly used in Ayurveda and integrative medicine are also classified as adaptogens due to their complex polymolecular profiles. Adaptogenic herbs have the 'intelligence' or chemical complexity to provide the body with a variety of benefits. The numerous compounds comprising adaptogenic herbs promote homeostasis and equilibrium of physiological functions, thereby assisting the body in resisting the detrimental effects of stress. Herb phytochemicals modulate a variety of processes, including hormone modulation and regulation of the hypothalamic-pituitary-adrenal axis, which influences stress responses. Therapeutic effects may be the result of synergistic combinations of multiple plant compounds; therefore, global approaches are the most effective for scientific investigations in this context.

Greater than the sum of its parts.

Synergy, or a synergistic effect, refers to the phenomenon whereby the effect of a combination of plant compounds is greater than the sum of the effects from the individual compounds. When a plant compound interacts with multiple receptor types, or multiple distinct molecules interact with multiple receptors to enhance the therapeutic effect, this is an example of synergy. In other instances, plant molecules may increase the bioavailability or alter the metabolic rate or excretion rate of other plant compounds. Positive examples of synergy include complementary mechanisms, such as the immunomodulation by multiple plant-derived compounds.

Ayurvedic herbal regimens

Ayurveda and other traditional systems of medicine utilize individualized herbal formulations to treat the digestive tract, the mind, the body's stamina, hormones, and frequently a chief complaint among patients. The therapeutic benefit of these herbal remedies may be attributable, at least in part, to the cooperative and supportive actions of our gut's microbial community. Ayurvedic and other medicinal herbs modulate the abundance and activities of our intestinal microbes, which act as our personal bioreactors to aid in the digestion, transformation, and assimilation of the food we consume.

Research on Ayurvedic herbs

Fascinated by the connection of Ayurveda and the gut, I have devoted a decade of research to understanding the mechanisms by which Ayurvedic medicines work through the application of microbiology and powerful genomics technologies. Our research team investigated the potential biological mechanisms of herbal medicines and identified potent effects on the gut microbiome in both human cohorts and *in vitro* laboratory models that simulate the gut environment. We observed that Ayurvedic herbs exert significant prebiotic effects on the microbiota of the human intestine. Prebiotics, as we have learned in previous chapters, are compounds that promote the growth and activity of the beneficial microorganisms that live within us and aid in the digestion and optimal utilization of our foods, dietary supplements, and medications. Prebiotics provide sustenance for our intestinal microbiome. In this way, our intestinal microbiome can be viewed as a personal bioreactor that produces a variety of complex compounds that regulate our health and wellbeing.

Interestingly, I observed that the Ayurvedic digestive formula, or *Agni* mix, can be eaten before or with meals and frequently improves digestion in an individual with a simple change. Thus, turmeric, ginger, black pepper, and long pepper (Ayurvedic common name: pippili) were tested by our lab for their effects on gastrointestinal flora. These spices were shown to be prebiotic, anti-inflammatory, and pathogen -repressive. Thus, culinary spices increased certain good gut bacteria and decreased some undesirable ones.

I wanted to understand how these therapeutic herbs and spices affect gut microbiome structure and function. We evaluated sugar digestion and key microbial metabolic pathways for short-chain fatty acid production using computer-based methods. Short-chain fatty acids, essential fermentation byproducts, affect the intestinal mucosa and neurological system. Thus, we sought to understand which components of herbs modulate gut microorganisms, which microbial species increase with herb or spice ingestion, and what gut community activities or functional changes are occurring.

Our laboratory model showed that the gut microbial changes in response to herb consumption are driven by glycosyl hydrolases, not the herb's sugar content. Glycosyl hydrolases, microbe-produced enzymes, help break down polysaccharides, complex carbohydrates in the diet. Without our microbial friends, we cannot digest these carbohydrates. Complex carbohydrates in human diets select for bacteria with the enzymes needed to breakdown diet-introduced sugars.

In our gut environment model, turmeric induced significant modifications in gut microbiota composition including a boost in the abundance of several butyrate-producing bacteria. Butyrate, a short-chain fatty acid, fuels gut epithelial cells that line the intestine, promotes immunological processes, and is neuroactive. Several herbs enhance propionate synthesis, which improves liver lipid metabolism.

In a randomized, double-blind, placebo-controlled pilot clinical trial, we found that the extensive repertoire of specialized glycosyl hydrolase enzymes encoded in the genomes of important health-promoting microbes in the genera *Bacteroides*, *Bifidobacterium*, *Alistipes*, and *Parabacteroides*, whose abundance was increased by turmeric, breaks down polysaccharide sugar components in turmeric root. These microorganisms liberate carbohydrates that fuel fermentative bacteria, such as a vast clade of key *Clostridium* species, which create health-promoting metabolites like short-chain fatty acids. Thus, these culinary spices may modify the gut microbiota and community metabolism, promoting health beyond digestion. These findings imply that healthy lifestyle choices, like cooking with a wide variety of spices or taking an Ayurvedic formula for digestion, may be beneficial for these reasons. Larger-scale human trials are needed to corroborate these findings.

Triphala is an herbal formulation consisting of three desiccated fruits that has numerous clinical applications ranging from gastrointestinal disorders to skin-related conditions. In addition to promoting rejuvenation, the complex composition of these fruits also promotes stamina and immunity in large populations, such as the very young and elderly. I was especially intrigued by the complexity of Triphala formulation's chemical profile and vast scope of its clinical utility, and I became committed to investigate its effects on intestinal microbiota. Our research team investigated the effects of triphala, slippery elm, and licorice on human intestinal microbes in a laboratory model of the gut. These botanicals are commonly prescribed for gastrointestinal health and conditions of the gut.

These three herbal medicines for the digestive system induced changes in approximately one-third of the human intestinal microbial species profiled and increased the abundance of probiotic bacteria, including *Bifidobacterium*, *Lactobacillus*, and *Bacteroides* species. This group of bacteria responsive to herbs included species that produced beneficial butyrate. Additionally, herb supplementation diminished the number of species classified as potential pathogens. Further, the herbs increased the relative abundance of microbes that degrade specific amino acids, the building blocks of proteins, such as tryptophan, which the brain converts to serotonin. The products of these tryptophan degradation reactions serve as signaling molecules that influence the gut and nervous system in a positive manner. Indeed, tryptophan degradation products together with butyrate represent two metabolites that positively influence leaky gut.

In the context of the gut-brain axis, herbal formulations targeting the mind in Ayurvedic treatment are of critical importance. Many of these nervine herbs, which are herbs with specific trophism for and support for the nervous system, are classified as nootropics, meaning they enhance the general function of the nervous system, for example by enhancing memory and focus. Kapikacchu, gotu kola, brahmi (*Bacopa*), shankhapushpi, frankincense (*Boswellia*), jatamansi, bhringaraj, guduchi, ashwagandha, and shatavari are among the most frequently administered Ayurvedic nervine herbs that improve memory, temperament, and other neurological functions. Due to their clinical utility and potential impact on the gut-brain axis, this class of botanicals piqued my interest and became the subject of our research efforts. Herb supplementation changed the abundance of more than half of the observed intestinal species, and the strongest modulators were bacopa, guduchi, bhringaraj, ashwagandha, and shankhapushpi.

These nervine herbs alter intestinal microbial short chain fatty acid synthesis pathways to enhance butyrate levels, according to bioinformatics predictions. Butyrate is known for positive effects on myriad aspects of host physiology, including nourishing the gut lining and signaling via the gut-brain axis. Jatamansi, guduchi, and bacopa were predicted to increase beneficial butyrate-producing gut bacteria.

In our personal gut bioreactor, many gut species coordinate herb metabolism. Our computer-based methods discovered networks of microbes that may work together to respond to Ayurvedic herbs or carbohydrates. Thus, Ayurvedic herbs modulate gut structure, function, and metabolism as the herbs partially reprogram community metabolism. The microbes collaborate and respond to the herbs in a coordinated manner. These metabolic changes in the gut microbiota may affect enteric nervous system signals and the gut-brain axis.

How Ayurvedic herbs work

In conclusion, while we are still discovering additional biological mechanisms by which Ayurvedic herbs work therapeutically, our research has demonstrated that herbs exert a substantial prebiotic effect and increase the growth and activity of beneficial microorganisms in our guts while potentially inhibiting bacteria that may be undesirable. Certain gastrointestinal microbes use specialized enzymes to release sugars from botanicals so that other microbial groups can produce post-biotics, such as short-chain fatty acids. Other gut bacteria degrade amino acids, which are subsequently converted into neurotransmitters to regulate gut-brain functions.

It appears that microbes function as complex communities that can synchronize their responses to herbs and herb metabolism. Microbes in the intestine degrade polymolecular botanicals to make constituents such as polyphenols more bioavailable, and they also produce health-promoting compounds such as neuroactive butyrate. Working as interdependent communities, microorganisms provide a plethora of capabilities and health benefits that we could never achieve by ourselves. The discovery of the prebiotic effects of medicinal herbs on the modulation of gut microbes and their subsequent production of health-promoting metabolites (post-biotics) has broadened our understanding of herbal medicine to include microbes as mediators of therapeutic effects. There is no true separation of species, but rather interaction, collaboration, and the exchange of information and resources within a connected community.

Given these recent discoveries, we may modify our view of how Ayurvedic herbs drive therapeutic benefit. Herb constituents are surely absorbed directly (with varied efficiency) for dissemination to target sites in the body, but now we also see that perhaps other constituents of herbs, not traditionally viewed as therapeutic, play an important role in modulating the gut microbiota and its post-biotic effects. A second important mechanism that is hypothesized to connect herb therapeutic benefit to the gut microbiota is the microbially mediated biochemical transformation of herb constituents that may increase their absorption and/or bioactivity. The scientific investigations aimed at revisiting ancient medicinal practices coupled with modern technologies and scientific approaches are exciting and likely to elevate, or re-elevate the use of Ayurvedic medicine as their long-assumed clinical benefits may be confirmed using modern scientific procedures.

According to an Ayurvedic proverb, "if diet is wrong, medicine is of no use. If diet is correct, medicine is of no need."

Chapter 16
The Gut and Ayurvedic Medicine: Perfect health begins in the gut

This chapter is both a mini primer on foundational Ayurvedic theory as well as an exploratory guide containing traditional Ayurvedic herbal, dietary, and lifestyle recommendations for the gut-related diseases presented in Part 2 of this work. Readers will learn foundational Ayurvedic concepts such as *Tridoshic* theory, root causes of disease, and specific Ayurvedic remedies utilized in clinical practice for the gut and gut disorders.

Both Western and traditional medicine agree that health and disease begin in the gut. In addition to prebiotics, probiotics, and diet, the use of traditional herbs and lifestyle medicine also helps to modulate the gut microbiota towards health and homeostasis. Evidence-based research on the effects of herbs and lifestyle medicine therapies is increasing; however, these areas are still highly underfunded and under-researched, especially in the context of the microbiome. Integrative medicine practices, such as Ayurveda and meditation, are popular, but their effects on human physiology are not yet fully understood. Nonetheless, Ayurvedic medicine has stood the test of time for over 5,000 years in India and offers natural remedies to both prevent and treat disease. It is also a medical system that complements and integrates well with Western therapies, especially as it relates to the gastrointestinal tract.

Ayurveda, a Sanskrit word that means the 'Science of Life' or the 'Science of Perfect Health', is the traditional system of personalized medicine originating in India that emphasizes disease prevention, health promotion, and the reversal of disease. In order to approach a cure for disease, the etiology or cause must be understood. Ayurveda examines both gross and subtle causes of disease, and unlike many Western approaches, it addresses the root cause and not just the symptoms of disease. Ayurvedic medicine examines the relationship between the individual patient and the environment. In this context, Ayurvedic doctors determine the constitutional nature of the patient, which is largely based on genetic data, the nature of the current imbalance, which is often lifestyle and environmentally based, and the nature of the proposed therapy in the context of the patient's environment. From this understanding, the Ayurvedic clinician seeks to apply holistic treatment that will move the patient from a state of disharmony, disease, and dysbiosis to a state of harmony, health, and homeostasis.

While Ayurveda notes that the primordial cause of disease is forgetting one's true nature, failure of the intellect to make wholesome choices, and deterioration due to time and motion, there are also three main causes of disease that are most relevant to classifying the pathology and treating the individual patient or patient type from an Ayurvedic perspective. These are the three *doshas* called *vata*, *pitta*, and *kapha*.

The *doshas* are forces that govern physiology and that, in excess or in imbalance, can lead to disease. Each individual holds a unique constitution or balance of these three *doshas* that is determined at conception and likely affects the expression of our genetic material. This original constitution has a great impact on activities such as our metabolic, digestive, and emotional tendencies. Generally speaking, *vata dosha* is made of air and ether and is the force responsible for motion; in excess, it can cause pain. *Pitta dosha* consists mostly of fire and a small amount of water and governs digestion and metabolism; in excess, it may lead to inflammation or fever. *Kapha dosha* is made of earth and water and is the force that provides structure, stability, and immune strength; in excess, it may lead to swelling, mucous, or weight gain.

From a cellular perspective, *vata dosha* is responsible for the absorption and circulation of nutrients as well as the excretion of waste products. *Pitta* governs nutrient metabolism and energy production. *Kapha* provides stability to the cell membranes and small intracellular structures, or organelles.

In addition to the aforementioned major symptoms of *doshic* imbalance, there are myriad symptoms that may be associated with imbalance in different individuals and that reflect the qualities associated with the *dosha*. Some other symptoms of *vata* disturbance include weight loss, insomnia, constipation, nervousness, confusion, and feeling cold. Additional symptoms of *pitta* imbalance include bleeding, yellowing, excess hunger or thirst, anger, burning sensations, and excessive sweating. Excess *kapha* may provoke nausea, congestion, depression, lethargy, and feelings of heaviness in the digestive tract or whole body.

Ayurvedic treatment seeks to manage these imbalances with the concept that things with similar qualities will increase each other, and opposites cancel each other out. This simply means that conditions of heat are treated with cold, dryness is treated with moisture, etc. This easy-to-apply system of disease management relies on five-sense therapies, or therapies that address the qualities of that which is entering through the five senses of the individual.

Ayurveda recognizes seven distinct types of tissues that create the body, and the *doshas* can invade and vitiate these tissues, which are called the *dhatus*. The invaded tissue can be increased or decreased by the *dosha*, which leads to the manifestation of symptoms. The seven tissues (*dhatus*) relate to the mucous membranes and fluids of the body (*rasa*); red blood cells and blood vessels (*rakta*); muscle, skin, and ligaments (*mamsa*); fat (*medas*); bones, hair, and nails (asthi); the nervous system (*majja*); and reproductive fluids (*shukra*).

Also important in this context is *ojas*, which is not really a tissue but the subtle life force energy of the human system that is generated from the digestion, transformation, and internal refinement of our food. Its levels correlate with the strength of the immune system. Conditions of low *ojas* often lead to disease due to deregulated immune function.

There is also the concept of *ama*, which refers to both gross and subtle toxins produced by the poor digestion of food, experience, and anything taken in through the five senses. *Ama*, or toxicity, can cause a number of issues, including partially or fully obstructing a *srota*, which is a gross or subtle channel. The gastrointestinal tract is an example of a gross channel, and the subtle channels correlate with the location of particular tissues. Thus, the imbalance of the *doshas* can lead to disease, and the tissues (*dhatus*) and channels (*srotas*) are the sites of disease manifestation. *Ama* will tend to form when *Agni*, or the digestive capacity, is not optimal.

Given the central importance of the gut and digestion in Ayurveda, *Agni* is a crucial concept and clinical focus. *Agni* is referred to as the digestive fire or the ability to digest, transform, and assimilate food properly without undesirable byproduct formation. Its state can be normal, high, low, or variable, depending on the actions of the doshas and our actions in our own lives. By overlaying the lens of Ayurveda with that of microbiology, I propose that the gut microbiome represents some of the activities of *Agni* such as digestion, metabolism, transformation, and assimilation. Certain features of the gut microbiome such as species that produce specialized glycosyl hydrolase enzymes to digest dietary polysaccharides thereby exhibit features of the fire element or digestive fire within the gastrointestinal tract. Therefore, the health and state of *Agni* are reflected in the health and state of the gut microbiome. Thus, by caring for the gut microbiome, you may also support *Agni*, and vice versa.

Ayurveda views disease as originating in the gastrointestinal tract. The digestive process influences the *doshas* within the body. The *doshas* have natural home sites where they reside under normal conditions of homeostasis within the gastrointestinal tract. However, when homeostasis is disturbed, such as when a person is living in disharmony with their constitution and the environment, the *doshas* can accumulate at their home sites. If homeostasis continues to be disturbed, the *doshas* will become aggravated and overflow into the circulatory system, which carries them throughout the body. The *doshas* then relocate to the weakest tissues of the body. Finally, disease will manifest and then diversify, differentiate, or even metastasize. Interestingly, it is during this final and very late stage of disease pathology that allopathic medicine first diagnoses disease and first seeks to treat it. Ayurveda would view this as a very late stage of disease and thus more difficult to treat successfully. Indeed, Ayurvedic medicine diagnoses disease at the first stage of the disease process, which is *doshic* accumulation, and thus seeks to intervene at the earlier stages of disease.

The goal of Ayurveda is to treat the root cause, which is the digestive system, as part of every treatment plan. Ayurvedic treatment plans often target the digestive system, circulatory system, and site of disease. Thus, the stages of the disease process viewed through the lens of Ayurvedic medicine are accumulation, aggravation, overflow, relocation, manifestation, and diversification.

The *doshas* have home sites in the gastrointestinal tract and are associated with specific tissues as sites of *dosha* relocation, manifestation, and diversification of disease. *Vata*, when exposed to dryness (like increases like), will

347

accumulate at its home site in the large intestine. When it relocates, *Vata* tends to settle into the nervous system, kidneys, and bones.

To pacify *Vata*, one must consume warm, heavy, moist foods and develop stable lifestyle routines. *Pitta*, when exposed to oiliness, will accumulate at its home site in the small intestine and tend to relocate to the liver, spleen, eyes, and blood. *Pitta* is pacified by the intake of cool, dry, and heavy foods and the adoption of regular routines. *Kapha* resides in the stomach and will relocate to the respiratory system as well as the fluids, muscle, fat, and reproductive fluids of the body. The alleviation of *kapha* occurs when it is exposed to dry, light, and mobile things as well as warm, dry foods and invigoration or spontaneity.

The digestive process influences the three *doshas* as food moves through the system. As a result, the *doshas* ebb and flow like tides in a rhythmic manner with a beginning, middle, and end. The process starts in the stomach (home of *kapha*), continues to the small intestine (home of *pitta*), and finishes in the large intestine (home of *vata*). As food passes through each home site, the *doshas* may increase or become aggravated. If one has digestive symptoms, it is helpful to note how long after eating those symptoms develop. This provides clues as to which *dosha* is likely contributing to the specific gastrointestinal issue. Symptoms occurring immediately after eating are likely due to *kapha*. Those 1-2 hours after eating are usually *pitta*-related. Symptoms greater than 3 hours after eating or on an empty stomach are due to *vata*.

It is beneficial to consume a diet that is harmonious with one's constitution as well as pacifying any imbalance. There is an Ayurvedic proverb that "if diet is incorrect, medicine is of no use. If diet is correct, medicine is of no need." Diet represents our greatest environmental exposure, especially in the context of our immune system, which is located mainly in the gut, the microbiome, which helps digest and transform our food, and the *doshas*. Proper diet and digestion are of the utmost importance for health and well-being.

Inflammatory Bowel Disease (IBD)

Ulcerative colitis and Crohn's disease are chronic inflammatory bowel diseases (IBD) that may have an autoimmune component. While ulcerative colitis involves genetic predisposition and commonly affects the colon, Crohn's disease primarily affects the small intestine but can occur at any location along the gastrointestinal tract. Allopathic treatment often relies on drugs to address inflammation and suppress the immune system; however, Ayurveda offers many complementary adjunct herbal and sensory treatments to reduce malabsorption, inflammation, and diarrhea associated with IBD.

IBD is primarily a *pitta* condition that can also be mixed with *vata* and/or *kapha*. The site of disease manifestation, the constitution of the individual, and particular *doshas* that are imbalanced are important considerations in the personalized treatment of IBD with Ayurvedic medicine. However, while personalized treatment with a practitioner is important, some general recommendations can be gleaned from Ayurveda.

In terms of diet, Ayurveda generally prefers a greater percentage of cooked compared to raw foods, and this would indeed hold true in the context of IBD. Cooked foods are much easier to digest compared to raw foods and tend to be less gas-promoting and gentler for an inflamed gut. In the context of a flare-up, Ayurveda would also suggest eating light or a short fast for a strong individual. Mung soup, which is strongly *pitta*-pacifying, can be taken post-fast to reintroduce food or in weak patients that cannot fast in order to rebuild digestive capacity or *agni*. Mung soup and dahl are very easy to digest and assimilate, thus supporting overall nutritional status and gut healing. Hot, spicy, and oily foods should be avoided.

Herbs such as slippery elm are used to support the mucous membranes lining the gut and prevent future flare-ups. Aloe Vera, *Ashwagandha*, Slippery Elm, and *Praval Pishti* may promote healing of ulcerations in the gut. A very powerful herb, comfrey leaf, helps with both bleeding and ulcerations but must only be used under the close supervision of a practitioner to monitor liver enzyme levels. The anti-inflammatory herbs *turmeric*, *guduchi*, and licorice are important. Licorice should only be taken short-term under a practitioner's care due to the possible development of hypertension or in the form of deglycyrrhizinated licorice (DGL) to reduce potential side effects. Cold infusions of the important gastrointestinal formulation *Triphala* can be taken long-term to support proper elimination and colon health in general. A cold infusion is adding the dried herb powder to room temperature water and allowing to sit a few hours or ideally overnight. This is a gentle steep that does not use hot water, but instead steeps gently over a longer period of time. Digestive aids such as ginger, nutmeg, fennel, and *asafoetida* are helpful for stabilizing digestion and absorption.

Lifestyle recommendations from Ayurveda include avoiding factors that increase *pitta* and *vata doshas*. For pacifying *pitta*, this balancing approach includes avoiding hot, oily, and spicy foods and activities that provoke hot emotions, especially anger. To pacify vata, the individual can avoid eating too many dry, light, or raw foods and allowing too many cold emotions such as anxiety and worry to dominate. If moods such as anger or anxiety are problematic, Ayurvedic herbs can be used that target the brain grossly and the *srota,* or channel, of the mind subtly. For anxiety and worry, nervine sedatives such as *Ashwagandha, Shankhapushpi,* and *Jatamansi* are often used together with nervine tonics such as *Ashwagandha* and *Gotu* Kola. For anger, cool nervine sedatives such as *Gotu Kola* and *Skullcap* are used with cool nervine tonics such as *Shatavari, Bacopa,* and *Shankhapushpi.* A portion of IBD patients may be highly reactive to stress. In such cases, stress-reducing practices such as meditation, yoga, breath work, and concentration-based activities can be incorporated daily.

Irritable Bowel Syndrome (IBS)

Irritable Bowel Syndrome (IBS) is a non-inflammatory disease of both intestines that causes alternating constipation and diarrhea with possible associated abdominal pain. The biological mechanisms and causes underlying IBS are not fully understood. Some researchers hypothesize that various types of stress, emotional factors, and food allergies may play a role. Whether food allergies are a cause or consequence of IBS is unknown. In addition, genes that correlate with an increased risk of developing allergic diseases might also contribute to the development of symptoms in some individuals.

Ayurveda defines IBS as a chronic imbalance characterized by high *vata* or *pitta.* In cases of increased *vata,* the individual will have gas, constipation, and abdominal pain. Alternating constipation and diarrhea are also possible. With high *pitta*, diarrhea and abdominal pain are usually present. *Kapha* may also be increased along with either *dosha*, and in such cases, mucous will be present in the stools. *Agni,* or digestive capacity, is also imbalanced according to the *dosha* that is affecting it. In *vata* cases, the digestive fire will be variable, and in *pitta* cases, it will be increased. However, if toxicity or *ama* is present, the digestive capacity will be low. Signs of *ama* include foul breath, tongue coating, fatigue, blemishes, indigestion, and weight gain. *Ojas,* or vital life force and immunity, are considered low in cases of IBS. Symptoms vary from person to person, often come and go, and may be accompanied by mood disorders. Stress or related psychological factors may play a role, and individuals are often highly susceptible to stress.

Dietary recommendations include avoiding any trigger foods, eating small meals, and monitoring for dehydration if diarrhea is present. A short period on a light diet or mung soup can help begin the process of rebuilding the digestive fire. A subsequent gradual reintroduction of easily digestible and properly spiced foods such as thicker soups, mung dahl with rice, and cooked vegetables should be followed for the proper restoration of *agni*. Heavier and oilier foods should be reintroduced only after digestive capacity has been restored. Once the digestive fire is rebalanced, a more nourishing diet should be consumed in order to rebuild tissues and *ojas*, which will increase tolerance to stress.

Herbs such as Slippery Elm, fresh Aloe Vera, and *Triphala* can be helpful for IBS, especially in cases of constipation. For constipation and gas, non-habit-forming laxatives such as *Triphala*, which gently increases peristalsis, can be used. Long-term use of bowel tonics such as Slippery Elm and cold infusions of *Triphala* (*shita kshaya*) is helpful in many cases. Demulcent herbs such as *shatavari* and licorice, which should only be taken short-term due to the possible development of hypertension, treat the underlying dryness. Carminatives such as ginger, *asafoetida*, and black pepper help reduce gas. If diarrhea or loose stools are present, demulcents such as *shatavari* and licorice and cool digestive aids such as fennel, cardamom, and coriander can be taken. Sage, nutmeg, and psyllium are also helpful for diarrhea. *Trikatu* is used when *ama,* or toxicity, is present. If mood disorders occur, the nervine sedatives and tonics suggested in the preceding section on IBD are recommended.

Lifestyle recommendations for IBS include activities that promote stress reduction and the building of *ojas*. Regular yoga, meditation, and breath work, or *pranayama,* can be employed to manage stress. *Ojas* can be increased with rest, oil therapies that incorporate massage techniques, and generally living a *sattvic* lifestyle, or one that is balanced and not overly stimulating to the five senses. Regular routines that include eating and sleeping at the same time should be adopted in order to stabilize *pitta* and *vata*. If signs of *ama* or toxicity are present, individuals can seek consultation at an Ayurvedic clinic for advice and candidacy regarding various types of *panchakarma*, which are Ayurveda's key protocols for cleansing and rejuvenation.

Obesity and Type 2 Diabetes Mellitus

Type 2 diabetes (T2D) results from abnormal insulin utilization and impaired blood sugar tolerance. It frequently occurs in overweight and obese children and adults. Excessively high blood sugar levels can lead to a coma. Long-term complications due to the resulting circulatory dysfunction affect areas such as the eyes, kidneys, nerves, and extremities. The primary cause of T2D is being overweight, and clinical data show that the condition is reversible using a lifestyle approach focusing on proper diet and exercise. Ayurveda interprets T2D as being caused by increased *kapha dosha*.

Ayurvedic dietary recommendations include a light diet that focuses on stabilizing blood sugar levels and supporting a healthy weight. The bitter taste is best for this purpose, and the pungent taste also helps with weight loss. Heavy, oily foods that increase *kapha*, such as meats and nuts, should be reduced. The sweet taste should also be minimized, especially simple sugars that are found in processed foods, milk, and fruits. Whole grains should be used in moderation, according to the individual. Overconsumption of meat, alcohol, milk products, and starch contributes to this condition. A plant-based diet is often supportive for most people with T2D.

An Ayurvedic approach primarily relies upon endocrine tonics and hypoglycemic herbs to target deregulated insulin and blood sugar, with bitters and anti-obesity herbs for weight gain. Additional herbs may also be used if complications such as neurological or cardiovascular dysfunction are present. Herbs for reducing blood sugar levels include *Bilva*, *Neem*, *Gurmar*, *Saptaranga*, and *Guggul* resin. *Shilajit* is a mineral that is both an endocrine tonic and a hypoglycemic. The anti-obesity herbs *Gurmar*, *Neem*, *Trikatu*, *Chitrak*, and *Guggul* resin are supportive in these cases. Strong bitters that also reduce *kapha* and encourage weight loss include *kutki*, *barberry*, and *gentian*.

Lifestyle recommendations include intensive exercise, which is evidence-based for reducing blood sugar, according to Strength. Excessive sleep, napping, and daytime sleep are not advised so as not to increase the quality of being heavy and stable. Instead of using oils, self-massage or body therapies can include dry herbal powders for greater purification and stimulation of the tissues. Sensory therapies focus on *kapha*-pacifying colors and essential oils that are usually warm, uplifting, and stimulating. Red, which correlates with the pungent taste, particularly encourages weight loss as it is the hottest and purifying color.

Leaky Gut, Food Allergy, and Inflammation

The evolving hypothesis and model of intestinal permeability or 'leaky gut' can be framed in the context of Ayurvedic principles to describe both pathology and disease reversal. Early symptoms include bloating and bowel changes, which may lead to signs of inflammation, which include fatigue, malaise, joint pain, and skin changes. It is hypothesized that leaky gut develops due to a cascade of inflammation from various insults to the gut mucosal lining that results in luminal contents such as pathogens and other microbial antigens, and products of poor digestion entering deeper tissues. In turn, an immune response is mounted, which increases inflammation that further disrupts the intestinal barrier, affects nutrient absorption, and may lead to food allergies. Food sensitivities and allergies promote additional inflammation. It is hypothesized that these immune responses may play a role in the development of certain types of autoimmune diseases, such as Hashimoto's. In addition, some naturopathic doctors suggest that signs of leaky gut include IBD, food allergies, autoimmunity, certain skin conditions, thyroid

357

disorders, malabsorption, mood issues, and even autism. The condition is complex and is not fully understood.

As digestion becomes impaired, *ama,* or toxicity, begins to accumulate, which interferes with normal functioning and can lead to other imbalances. The inflammation in this condition is due to increased *Pitta* in the digestive system, specifically the subdosha *Pachaka Pitta* in the small intestine. High *Pitta* can then disturb *Agni*, the digestive fire, such that food is poorly digested. Partially digested food further irritates a weakened mucosal lining and is considered ama, or toxicity, in Ayurveda. Any malabsorption is a result of increased *Vyana Vayu* (circulation of nutrients) and *Samana Vayu* (absorption of nutrients), both *subdoshas* of *Vata*. In general, *vata* governs the movement of molecules across cell membranes. Patients with intestinal permeability may have low *Ojas,* or subtle life energy, and those that develop autoimmune conditions are very likely to have low *Ojas*.

The lens of Ayurveda can frame leaky gut as a primary *Pitta* imbalance with possible secondary *Vata* vitiation, variable *Agni*, and possible low *Ojas*. Dietary recommendations include a short period on a light diet or, ideally, mung soups and Ayurvedic *kitcheree* made of dahl and rice with cooling spices such as coriander, fennel, and cardamom to rebuild the digestive fire. A slow reintroduction of easily digestible foods and foods prepared with cooling *Pitta*-lowering digestive spices, such as thicker soups, mung dahl with rice, and well-cooked vegetables, should be followed for the proper restoration of *Agni*. Heavier and oilier foods are reintroduced slowly. Once the digestive fire is rebalanced, a more nourishing, *Pitta*-lowering diet should be consumed in order to increase *Ojas*.

Healthy fats such as avocado, coconut oil, and ghee help nourish the colon and should be favored in the diet. Ghee, or clarified butter, contains butyric acid and is a very helpful addition to meals. The gut microbiota converts fiber and starch into the short-chain fatty acid butyric acid, which provides nutrition to the cells lining the gut and provides signaling to the brain via the vagus nerve. Ghee helps normalize *Agni,* which is necessary for proper digestion and absorption as well as the building of healthy *Dhatu,* or tissue, and O*jas*. Ghee may also provide mood-stabilizing signals to the parasympathetic nervous system that are needed in times of gut dysbiosis. Vegans can use coconut oil as a substitute for ghee because it has similar cooling properties to ghee. A gut that is nourished with oils will have increased barrier integrity and immunity. Simple sugars, processed foods, fried foods, and food triggers should be avoided. Depending on your diet, bone broth, fermented dairy and vegetables, wild-caught fatty fish, high-potency multi-strain probiotics such as Progurt's human isolates, flax seeds, and well-cooked fruits and vegetables are also beneficial for gut nourishment and to promote repair. Digestive spices such as turmeric, ginger, cumin, fenugreek, coriander, fennel, and cinnamon should be taken with foods for proper digestion and assimilation. Since the gut and brain are connected via a bidirectional communication network and more, gut repair may improve mood or behavioral imbalances.

An Ayurvedic herbal approach may include anti-inflammatories, demulcents, *dipanas* (digestives), and hepatoprotective plants. Anti-inflammatories such as turmeric, ashwagandha, guduchi, licorice, and amla can be used. To improve the integrity of the gut mucosal lining, demulcents or demulcent herbs followed by some astringents are often useful. Demulcent plants used to improve the gut epithelium include aloe vera, Marshmallow root, Slippery Elm, and Licorice root. Licorice root is an adaptogenic herb and demulcent that may help reduce cortisol levels, improve stomach acid production, and maintain the mucosal lining of the stomach and duodenum. In cases of leaky gut, liver-supporting herbs such as Bhumyamalaki, Guduchi, Barberry, Turmeric, and Milk Thistle are also helpful to reduce inflammation and promote adequate detoxification. Integrative approaches incorporate supplements such as probiotics, digestive enzymes, L-glutamine, and quercetin to support the intestinal lining and reduce permeability.

Ayurvedic lifestyle recommendations include daily stress reduction techniques. Stress is a known culprit involved in many chronic gastrointestinal diseases and should be reduced as a focus. Yoga, meditation, or other mind-body contemplative practices should be practiced daily. The avoidance of any potential food triggers, environmental toxins, excess antibiotic use, excess sugars, processed foods, industrial oils, and certain medications that affect the gut lining, such as long-term ibuprofen or aspirin, is suggested. An assessment from a *Panchakarma* specialist to design a custom program to target the removal of *Ama* and the subsequent restoration of *Ojas* is highly recommended. *Panchakarma* is the most powerful detoxification and rejuvenation protocol practiced in Ayurvedic medicine and is offered by specialists, ideally in a residential retreat setting.

Celiac Disease

Celiac disease is a small intestinal disease with a genetic predisposition that can lead to gluten sensitivity. Gluten, a component of wheat and other grains, triggers an immune response that leads to damage of the small intestinal villi and, in turn, malabsorption and secondary pathologies. Stress and a poor diet also contribute to the development of disease. Patients often present with gas and bloating, abdominal cramps, weight changes, alternating constipation and diarrhea, malaise, and skin issues. Possibly due, at least in part, to genetic factors, this condition often presents with other autoimmune diseases. Without proper medical diagnosis and treatment, this condition can lead to serious health issues.

Ayurvedic medicine interprets the pathology as a dual-*doshic Vata/Pitta* imbalance with variable *Agni,* or digestive fire, and possible low *Ojas.* There is variable digestion (*Vata*), malabsorption (*Vata*), and inflammation (*Pitta*) of the intestinal villi. If there is mucous in the stools, Kapha is also vitiated; the condition is tri-doshic in nature, and all three *doshas* must be reduced. An Ayurvedic approach focuses on gastrointestinal symptoms, weight loss, malabsorption, and inflammation.

Ayurvedic dietary recommendations focus on the avoidance of gluten and gluten-containing foods. Adherence to a *Vata-Pitta*-pacifying diet or tri-doshic diet (if necessary) will help reduce gastrointestinal symptoms as well. The best taste is the sweet taste, which favors heavier foods. This must be done without overeating, eating too many carbohydrates, or otherwise overwhelming an already unstable *Agni* or digestive fire. Sweet foods include nuts, seeds, meats, rice, quinoa, amaranth, dairy, some vegetables, berries, fruits, and ghee. The hot, light, and dry qualities must be reduced, so foods that are warm or a bit cool, heavy, and slightly oily are best. The salty, pungent, and bitter tastes are the least beneficial due to their drying nature, and they are thought to be eaten only rarely during times of imbalance. A tri-*doshic* diet reduces the intake of food that has the qualities of being hot, heavy, and dry. All tastes are used, but in moderation and with proper spices such as cardamom, coriander, cumin, fennel, saffron, and turmeric. Ghee and dipana (digestive spices) should be added to the diet to stabilize *Agni*.

An Ayurvedic approach favors the use of *dipanas* (digestive herbs and spices), nutritive tonics, and anti-inflammatories. Ayurvedic herbs for the treatment of associated gas, bloating, and poor digestion include *dipanas* (digestives) such as *asafoetida*, ginger, black pepper, fennel, and cumin. For weight loss, nutritive tonics such as *Ashwagandha*, *Shatavari*, and Slippery Elm are often implemented. The inflammation is treated with herbs such as turmeric, ashwagandha, guduchi, and licorice.

Lifestyle recommendations focus on stress identification and reduction. The patient can seek to identify particular stressors and frame them in the context of the *doshas*, such as *Vata* or *Pitta*. With such knowledge, the patient can modify their behavior and types of sensory input to pacify the primary *dosha* involved. To reduce the *ama,* or toxicity, that builds up due to poor digestion and plan for the rebuilding of Ojas, an assessment from a *Panchakarma* specialist is recommended for Celiac patients interested in Ayurveda.

Conclusion

To approach a cure for a disease, it is necessary to comprehend its etiology or cause. Ayurveda analyzes both gross and subtle causes of disease, and unlike many Western approaches, it focuses on the root cause rather than merely the symptoms. Ayurvedic medicine investigates the relationship between the patient and the surrounding environment. According to Ayurveda, disease originates in the digestive tract. Indeed, Ayurvedic medicine diagnoses disease at the earliest stage of the disease process and thus attempts to intervene earlier in the development of the disease, when it is most easily treated.

According to an Ayurvedic proverb, "if diet is incorrect, medicine is of no use. If diet is correct, medicine is of no need." Diet represents our greatest environmental exposure, particularly in relation to our immune system, which is primarily located in the gut, and the microbiome, which aids in the digestion and transformation of our food. Ayurveda emphasizes that diet and digestion are crucial for health and well-being. To support a healthy gut microbiome, we must consume a wide diversity of fruits, vegetables, herbs, and culinary spices and take measures to improve our digestion. With knowledge of tools to feed, support, and nourish our gut, we can rest assured that we are on a path to better health.

It could be that those individuals who are non-responders to herbal medicine treatment are lacking microbes that contain the enzymatic functions necessary to break down the sugars in the herbs themselves.

Chapter 17
Preventative Medicine: An Ounce of Prevention with Ayurvedic Diet, Herbs, and Lifestyle

This chapter serves as a brief introduction to preventative medicine using the dietary and lifestyle techniques of Ayurveda. The novel impact of Ayurvedic herbs on the gut microbiome is addressed. Ayurvedic daily dietary and lifestyle routines are later explored as prevention to facilitate a long-lasting quality of life.

Ayurveda is a system of medicine that treats the whole individual, and because it is personalized medicine, and perhaps the first personalized system of medicine, it is imperative to work with a qualified Ayurvedic practitioner or integrative medicine provider with training in Ayurveda. Nonetheless, the purpose of this chapter is to introduce and orient inquisitive readers to seasonal, circumstantial, and other approaches to holistic prevention methods.

Ayurvedic medicinal herbs.

In terms of medicinal herbs, four core personalized formulations targeting digestion, or *agni*, the mind, stamina, hormones, and a chief complaint, if present, often constitute a base herb regimen. Since health begins in the gut, digestive herbs are arguably the most important. These are often culinary spices that can be used in cooking. As mental disturbances lead to stress-related disorders, the mind formula should also be taken diligently. These formulas should be personalized and change based on the individual's needs.

Ayurvedic herbs, and medicinal herbs in general, modulate the composition and activities or functions of our microbes. Our research has revealed the especially potent effects of Ayurvedic herbs on the gut microbiome in both humans and in laboratory models that mimic the gut environment. Ayurvedic herbs exert prebiotic effects on gut microbial communities, suggesting that the activities of microbes in the gut may play an important role in the medicinal properties of medicinal herbs like those from Ayurveda.

Herbs to support digestive fire.

Turmeric is often used in the core digestion-promoting, or *agni,* formulation, which is a cornerstone of the Ayurvedic lifestyle, as well as therapy taken just before or with meals. Turmeric is used liberally as a culinary spice in Ayurvedic cooking and food therapy to support digestion and absorption. It is also used as a medicinal herb. Thus, our research group was interested in how this important herb and one of its key constituents affect the gut microbes in healthy humans.

In a randomized, double-blind clinical trial, our lab examined the effects of *Curcuma longa* (common name: turmeric) with piperine (derived from black pepper often added to turmeric or curcumin supplements for improved absorption), curcumin (one of the biologically active constituents of turmeric) with piperine extract, and placebo on the gut microbiome in a small cohort of healthy subjects. After 8 weeks of dietary supplementation, it was observed that turmeric-treated subjects displayed a modest 7% increase in the number of observed species posttreatment, while individuals taking curcumin displayed an average increase of 69% in detected species. This gut microbiome response was highly personalized and featured both responders and non-responders to dietary supplement treatment.

In the context of many dietary therapies, it is observed that there will be responders and non-responders to treatment, and this phenomenon is not well understood. It should be emphasized that responders and non-responders in this context refer to effects on the gut microbiota and do not necessarily refer to response to the herb itself. It could be that those individuals who are non-responders to herbal medicine treatment are lacking microbes that contain the enzymatic functions necessary to break down the sugars in the herbs themselves. In addition, the responders to treatment had a similar or concordant pattern of response within both the curcumin- and turmeric-treated groups. Thus, it is possible that curcumin could represent a driving factor for most of the changes observed in the turmeric-supplemented individuals.

In all the groups, gut microbiota displayed significant variation over time and an individualized response to treatment. This observation highlights the dynamic flux of our microbiome that is happening all the time in response to our lifestyle as well as their greatest environmental exposure, which is what we eat. As this was a small pilot study, larger clinical trials seeking to confirm these results and dive deeper into biological mechanisms are warranted.

As digestive formulation is a key aspect of the Ayurvedic diet and little is known about their impact on gut microbes, I was also interested in exploring more deeply the impact of culinary spices used in this context. In one study, our lab used a laboratory model of the gut environment by applying *in vitro* anaerobic cultivation of human gut microbes to study the microbial modulatory effects of four culinary spices used to support digestive capacity: *Curcuma longa* (turmeric), *Zingiber officinale* (ginger), *Piper longum* (pippali or long pepper), and *Piper nigrum* (black pepper). These plants are also used as medicinal herbs, and thus there is a spectrum of culinary and medicinal herbs that may overlap. These spices all exhibited strong modulatory effects with both prebiotic effects and repressive effects of microbes that can be inflammatory (e.g., some of the beneficial microbes increased and some undesirable microbes decreased in the lab model).

Accordingly, I wanted to know more about what components of these culinary spices and medicinal herbs might be driving the gut microbes to change their growth rates and functional activities. Using a highly accurate measuring technique called mass spectrometry, we were able to use *in situ* or computer-based methods called genome reconstruction to examine the relevant sugar digestion pathways as well as key microbial metabolite pathways called short-chain fatty acids (SCFA). Short-chain fatty acids are important microbial products of fermentation that have widespread effects, including affecting the gut lining and the nervous system, as discussed previously. Thus, we sought to understand what aspects of the herbs are driving the effects on gut microbes, what microbes are changing in response to the herb or spice intake, and what activities or functional changes are happening within the gut community, which can be thought of as our own personal bioreactor.

Our *in vitro* results examining these culinary spices showed that the sugar composition of the herb itself is not the main driver of the gut microbial changes associated with herb intake, but the conserved functions of a gene family called glycosyl hydrolases are more strongly associated with herb response. Glycosyl hydrolases are enzymes that are encoded in microbial genomes to help break down complex sugars called polysaccharides. The presence of these complex sugars in our diet provides selective pressure on gut microbial communities such that microbes that contain the type of enzyme needed to break down the particular complex sugar introduced via the diet will grow by expanding their numbers and activities.

While the herbs contain amino acids as well as sugars, based on the data, we conclude that the digestion of herbs by gut communities primarily involves sugar fermentation as a dominant prebiotic force, whereas amino acid fermentation was considered a minor contributor. Among the culinary spices analyzed in our laboratory model with human stool samples, only turmeric promoted changes in gut microbiota composition that are predicted to increase butyrate-producing taxa. Thus, these spices may drive beneficial changes in gut microbiota to alter their community or collective metabolism to promote salubrious effects on digestion. Our study should be followed up in a human cohort to confirm these findings and understand how herb metabolism contributes to both known and unknown health benefits.

Interestingly, evidence that turmeric positively impacts leaky gut has been reported, despite it well established poor solubility. This finding helps to clarify a long-standing paradox associated with turmeric and curcumin. Many studies have demonstrated the systemic effects of these medicinal herbs on human physiology despite very low measurable quantities of these herb constituents in the bloodstream. The activity of turmeric and curcumin that restores proper gut permeability may help to resolve this apparent discrepancy, as the beneficial systemic effects of these herbs may stem largely from the therapeutic effects of reduced gut permeability.

An extraordinary herbal formulation for the gut

Triphala is a commonly used and clinically studied herbal formulation of three dried fruits with many clinical applications in Ayurveda and contains a combination of *Terminalia bellerica* (common name: bibhitaki) and *Terminalia chebula* (common name: haritaki). In Ayurveda, it is considered a cornerstone treatment for gastrointestinal disorders ranging from constipation to colitis and is used for a variety of gut and skin-related conditions. In addition, the complexity of these rejuvenation-promoting fruits allows them to be employed for many applications, including long-term usage for stamina and immunity support as well as in the very young and elderly.

Our lab group was interested in the potential gut microbiota modulatory effects of Triphala in healthy humans, so we conducted a 4-week randomized, double-blind, placebo-controlled pilot clinical trial for a closer look. Our group also included another medicinal herb used to treat gut and skin conditions called *Rubia cordifolia* (common name: manjistha). Thus, we had 3 treatment groups: a Triphala-treated, Manjistha-treated, and placebo-treated group to compare the effects of a 4-week course of dietary supplementation.

We observed that the gut microbiota responses were very personalized, and neither herbal medicine uniformly altered species in test subjects. The subjects in both groups that received Ayurvedic herbs showed a trend of decreased Firmicutes to Bacteroidetes ratios and an increase in the relative abundance of *Akkermansia muciniphila*. While these are pilot data that should be confirmed in larger clinical trials, it is interesting to note that Firmicutes are often generally associated with negative impacts on glucose and fat metabolism, with increased Firmicutes to Bacteroidetes ratios associated with obesity and type 2 diabetes. Similarly, low levels of *Akkermansia* are correlated with obesity. Thus, larger trials examining the therapeutic impact of these herbs on the gastrointestinal tract and beyond in humans are warranted.

Given our interest in medical herbs that target the gut, our lab also examined a few commonly prescribed herbs for gastrointestinal health in our laboratory model. In the study, we investigated the effects of *Ulmus rubra* (common name: slippery elm) and *Glycyrrhiza glabra* (common name: licorice), and triphala on gut microbes derived from humans in our laboratory model of the gut. We observed profound changes in diverse gut species with herb supplementation, with each herb driving unique community formations with discrete effects. In fact, all three herbal medicines induced changes in about 1/3 of the human gut species profiled and increased the abundance of many bacteria known to promote human health, such as *Bifidobacterium* spp., *Lactobacillus* spp., and *Bacteroides* spp. This included increasing species that produce beneficial butyrate. The herb supplementation also reduced the abundance of species deemed potential pathogens, such as *Citrobacter freundii* and *Klebsiella pneumoniae*.

Herbal medicines for digestion induced blooms of butyrate- and propionate-producing species and increased the abundance of glycosyl hydrolase families induced by each herbal medicine. Licorice, which is the sweetest herb of the three examined in this set of herbs, interestingly increased the abundance of several glycosyl hydrolase families. Thus, the profound prebiotic potential of medicinal herbs suggest that the therapeutic benefits are due, at least in part, to the modulatory actions on gut microbiota that promote healthy colonic function and absorption, reduced inflammation, and protection from opportunistic infection.

Herbs for the nervous system and mind

In addition to the digestive formula, the mind formulas used in Ayurveda is of key importance. Many of these nervine herbs, which are herbs that specifically support the nervous system or otherwise target the system, are classified as nootropics, meaning that they improve the function of the neurological system. Given that research on the neurological effects of medicinal herbs on human gut microbes is scarce, we used our laboratory model of the gastrointestinal tract with Ayurvedic herbs and human gut microbes to learn more. We expanded our strategy to include analysis of the predicted sugar utilization of the gut microbes with a very accurate technique called quantitative mass spectrometry to measure the sugar content of the herbs and thus discern potential drivers of the gut microbe community changes induced by the medicinal herbs.

We investigated 10 commonly prescribed Ayurvedic nervine herbs that improve memory, mood, and other functions, namely, kapikacchu, gotu kola, brahmi (*Bacopa*), shankhapushpi, frankincense (*Boswellia*), jatamansi, bhringaraj, guduchi, ashwagandha, and shatavari. Herb supplementation induced profound changes in many diverse gut species; in fact, 77% of detected species were altered in abundance by herb supplementation. Bacopa, guduchi, bhringaraj, ashwagandha and shankhapushpi were the most potent modulators examined. In addition, 56% of detected species were altered in abundance by more than 100-fold by at least 1 nervine herb.

Ashwagandha, bhringaraj, guduchi and kapikacchu-supplementation increased the abundance of several beneficial *Bifidobacterium* and *Bacteroides* species, while shatavari promoted growth of several beneficial *Bacteroides* species that are dominant members of the gut. Kapikacchu induced the growth of an important microbe, *Ruminococcus bromii,* which helps degrade dietary fibers and resistant starch in our diet. Interestingly, brahmi/bacopa, ashwagandha, and kapikacchu promoted the growth of a dominant member of the gut community, namely *B. thetaiotaomicron*. This gut microbe makes polysaccharide A, which is a substance that stimulates inflammation-suppressing regulatory T cells in the gut. Bacopa promoted the growth of several beneficial and dominant members of the gut such as Bacteroides species.

These nervine herbs were predicted to modulate SCFA metabolite production pathways in gut microbes to potentially increase levels of neuroactive butyrate. Several of the herbs, including jatamansi, guduchi, and bacopa selected for increased abundance of butyrate-producing gut microbes. In addition, many gut species were identified by co-occurrence network analyses in terms of response coordination to herb supplementation. This analysis revealed networks of microbes that may work together in the presence of certain herbs or sugars. Thus, the nervine herbs demonstrate strong modulatory action on the gut microbiota in terms of its structure and metabolism. These changes in the metabolism of the community may affect signaling in the enteric nervous system and ultimately the gut-brain axis, although future studies in human cohorts are required to confirm such speculation. This knowledge of how Ayurvedic herbs function not only informs future research developments but also motivates us to adopt these evidence-based supplements for gut health.

Ayurvedic medicine offers many easy and natural ways to improve your digestion with lifestyle changes. Recall that Ayurveda is a Sanskrit term meaning "science of perfect health" and literally translates as "knowledge of life," which is knowledge about how to live a healthy, happy life. Ayurveda seeks to bring us back into balance by providing guidelines for living in harmony with nature's rhythms so that the underlying wisdom of the body can naturally promote the reestablishment of health and homeostasis. Ayurveda helps us move from disharmony, dysbiosis, and disease to harmony, homeostasis, and health. In the next section, we will explore some wisdom from Ayurveda on eating and daily lifestyle routines.

Ayurvedic eating tips

Most Americans suffer from mild digestive disturbances such as constipation, gas, bloating, diarrhea, heartburn, and heaviness after eating, and many endure more serious conditions. Ayurvedic medicine interprets the mild digestive disturbances as warning signs from the body that imbalance has begun and thus seeks to intervene at this very early stage of disease to prevent the manifestation of disease. Ayurveda offers simple remedies that are healthy lifestyle changes that can be easily practiced at home. Ayurveda focuses on what food is eaten, when food is eaten, and how food is eaten.

Both what we eat and what we actually digest and absorb are equally important. This is important given that the state of our gut and physiology will determine how much we digest and absorb and, thus, how much we benefit from what we eat. Those suffering from digestive disturbances are not obtaining the full benefit of the nutrients in the food that they are eating; new bodily tissues are built less strong and healthy, and undigested food particles can lead to inflammation and gut dysbiosis.

In terms of what you eat, care should also be taken to eat fresh, whole, and, if possible, organic foods. It may be useful to think about eating for your microbiome. The microbiome wants a wide variety of soluble fiber, insoluble fiber, and starch, including beans, vegetables, spices, and edible herbs. Eat for your imbalance or focus on your constitutional balancing if you have not yet found a practitioner to help you properly identify imbalances. Remember that Ayurveda is for everyone, including vegans or those on special diets; thus, in such cases, one can use substitutes with items containing similar qualities, such as coconut oil (vegan) for ghee (dairy).

Importantly, how you eat also plays a key role in determining what you will digest and assimilate. The act of eating is both spiritual and life-sustaining. The food we take into our bodies will be broken down and used as building blocks for new parts of our bodies. It is a spiritual process in that the molecules in the food have been around since the beginning of time, recycling and thus connecting us to all that ever was, is, and will be. From this perspective, we can begin to perceive eating as a meditative or contemplative experience, which also calms the body and ensures healthy digestion.

Here are some Ayurvedic Guidelines for Healthy Eating to help improve your digestion, absorption of nutrients, and elimination through guidance on how and when to eat:

1. Eat only when you are hungry. This ensures that your prior meals have been digested, so that your new meal will be digested and absorbed without the formation of any toxins from undigested food particles.

2. Eat food in a calm setting. Your environment can help or interfere with your digestion, especially if you are eating on the go, standing up, in the car, or in a chaotic environment. Ideally, find a calm space that is free of clutter and contains some beauty. Some ideas include clearing the table of items and adding some fresh wildflowers or a colorful table runner. Sit down to eat.

3. Eat without distractions. When the mind is distracted, food is often chewed improperly. If you must eat in the car, pull over to eat. Put your devices away and shift your focus to the experience of eating and chewing thoroughly to support digestion.

4. Take three deep breaths before you eat. This time allows you to stop your activity, which interferes with digestion, relax, and connect mindfully to your food. This can also serve as an opportunity to say a prayer or affirmation or take some additional moments of silence in gratitude for the food itself and those who brought it to you.

5. Eat with a peaceful mindset. It is best to be in a peaceful state of mind for optimal digestion. If you choose to speak with others, keep the conversation light and avoid heated topics such as politics. Feeling very stressed, angry, or otherwise disturbed while eating will interfere with key digestive processes. Thus, skip the meal or meditate first if you are feeling very agitated during mealtime.

6. Food should be eaten warm. Ayurveda recommends that most of your food be served warm since cooking makes food more easily digested and absorbed. Cold foods weaken the digestive fire, which can lead to the formation of toxins from undigested food. A Western scientific interpretation of this concept relates to the fact that enzymes such as digestive enzymes tend to be more efficient at warmer temperatures.

7. Do not drink cold beverages and take only a little liquid with meals. As mentioned, temperature matters in terms of the efficiency of digestive

enzymes, so be sure to steer clear of cold drinks or ice with meals. Ideally, do not eat or drink anything straight out of the refrigerator. Drinks also weaken the digestive fire by diluting the digestive enzymes with liquid. Taking 1 cup of warm or room-temperature water with meals, if needed, is ideal. Wait at least 1-2 hours after eating before drinking larger quantities.

8. Chew, chew, chew. Chew food to an even consistency. Digestion begins in your mouth as salivary enzymes are released. Ayurveda also teaches that the six tastes are important for balancing our health, and interestingly, Western science has discovered taste receptors similar to those on the tongue within our gastrointestinal tract.

9. Eat food that is oily or moist. Oily and moist foods provide more nourishment to the body compared to dry foods, which are difficult to digest and eliminate. Food that is overly oily is also difficult to digest; thus, food should be moderately oily or moist.

10. Eat only until you are 2/3 to 3/4 full. This one can be quite a challenge, especially when delicious food is in front of you, but it is worth practicing. Overeating overwhelms the digestive system and enzymes and leads to poorly digested food and toxicity. Ayurveda suggests eating until you are

no longer hungry but satisfied. Anti-aging science also tells us that an easy way to extend our lives and promote healthy aging is to eat less. Another major benefit is that the mind and body will feel much lighter after eating.

11. Rest after meals. It is common to go right back to activity after eating. However, this productivity and movement interfere with digestion and our bodies' ability to stay in "rest and digest' mode. We want to rest for at least a few minutes after eating for maximum absorption of nutrients. One hour is ideal, according to Ayurveda; however, even 15 minutes of rest will provide much benefit. Another trick is to lie on your left side for 15 minutes to allow your digestive juices to pool and increase the rate of digestion.

12. Don't eat late. Try not to eat after sunset. Eating late negatively impacts our digestion, sleep, and metabolism. Finish eating a few hours before going to bed, and ideally go to bed by 10 PM.

13. Your Ayurvedic practitioner or other integrative clinician can also prescribe digestive herbs and diet per your unique constitution in a personalized way to target your unique digestive make-up as well as any imbalances. It is always recommended to approach Ayurveda with a practitioner to expertly personalize your treatment plan. In addition to knowing how to

eat, knowing when to eat and when not to eat is also vital for digestive health, and your practitioner can also advise you on this aspect of eating.

For best results, slowly incorporate 1 or 2 changes at a time into your daily regimen. This will prevent you from feeling overwhelmed by change and ensure that the changes you make are sustainable. Individuals often report significant improvements in digestion and elimination after incorporating even one of these changes consistently. For example, some people report less bloating after giving up cold drinks, while others report less constipation after eating until they are 75% full. It is well worth slowly working towards eating this way, given the abundant returns.

Ayurvedic lifestyle tips

According to Ayurveda, the three pillars of health are food, sleep, and sex. These should be taken in proper quantities, of proper qualities, at proper times, and in the right ways given the constitution and any imbalance experienced by an individual. An introduction to some of the common types of lifestyle therapies used in Ayurveda is described below.

Meditation is perhaps the most important component of Ayurvedic living and therapy. Practicing some form of meditation or mindfulness for at least 20 minutes first thing in the morning, in the evening as a transition to evening activities, and/or right before bed are often useful times. For new meditators and seasoned practitioners alike, there are supportive apps that can be used for training, such as the Insight Timer App, to assist with guided *Vipassana* meditation, although any type of guided support or not using support at all will be sufficient. Work towards a daily practice of consistent meditation.

Yoga postures and breathing exercises called pranayama are often also incorporated as lifestyle support in Ayurveda. These can be chosen based on the constitution and any imbalances in the individual. For example, forward-bending postures are grounding, while backbends can be slightly stimulating. Alternate nostril breathing is balancing, while rapid breathing, or 'breath of fire," is stimulating. These qualities are taken into account in the context of the person, the season of the year, and other factors to choose the best routine to promote homeostasis and ease.

Sleep is a pillar of health, per Ayurveda. Sleep hygiene and evening routines are fundamentally important for health and are known to impact the microbiome, yet subtleties are sometimes overlooked. Aim to go to bed by 10 p.m. Meditate again briefly in bed, then lay down and transition effortlessly to sleep. Be sure there are no lights or blue lights in the room. Keep the room dark (use curtains or an eye mask, no digital clocks or devices if you can) and cool.

Several self-care lifestyle therapies are often incorporated into Ayurvedic routines. For example, *Abhyanga,* as a self-oil massage prior to showering, can be grounding and nourishing for the body. Use warmed (on the stove in a double boiler for a minute) oil and apply. Then, use quick, long friction strokes on the long bones and circular strokes on the joints. Use oil on the face and focus massage on areas of concern to combat dryness.

Neti, or nasal irrigation, with a natural salt is another technique used in the morning for mental clarity and to reduce the effects of allergens and pollution. The practice of *neti* is often followed later with *nasya,* or the oiling of the nasal passages with medicated herbal oil. This nourishes and further protects the mucosal lining in the nostrils. Note that irrigation is later followed by oiling, as is often the case in Ayurveda. Ayurveda tends to seek balance, so rather than only applying a cleansing practice such as irrigation, a rejuvenating practice with oil often follows.

Another useful daily cleansing practice is *Chakshu Dhauti,* or eye washing, for tired, fatigued, or dry eyes. This can be done with organic rose water, which doubles as a facial toner spray, or a homemade filtered, cooled and filtered

389

Triphala hot water decoction by filling an eye cup. Eye cups come in plastic or glass and can be found online or at drug stores. Do gentle eye exercises for as long as is comfortable—about 30 seconds per eye or so. This helps with irritated and dry eyes.

For the health of the oral cavity, which has far-reaching effects, tongue scraping and oil pulling are highly effective for hygiene and gum care. Metal tongue scrapers can be used prior to brushing to remove bacterial buildup and reduce bad breath. Oil pulling by swishing for 20 minutes with coconut oil or a medicated oil removes bacteria under the gumline and nourishes the gums, oral cavity and cheeks.

Deep, slow abdominal breathing is one of the most effective methods to stimulate the optimal functioning of the vagus nerve, which regulates heart rate, stimulates the intestines, and activates the immune system. Changes in intraabdominal pressure from breath, certain movements like Yoga, or the use of yogic locks, or *bandhas*, are other ways to maintain vagus nerve health.

Vagus nerve stimulation techniques include:

Breathe slowly and deeply. Work towards a breath practice of six breaths per minute. Inhale deeply from the abdomen. As you inhale, visualize your abdomen expanding and your rib cage expanding. Exhale for a longer duration than you inhale. Exhalation initiates the relaxation response.

Other types of deep breathing, especially yogic *pranayama* practices, are also valuable. Humming is known to stimulate the vagus nerve, and the yogic *Bhramari*, or buzzing bee breath, is a powerful option that is both a breath practice and humming exercise. After a deep inhalation, close your ears with your fingers and make a buzzy, humming sound on exhalation for each round of breath.

Increasing intraabdominal pressure with yoga postures or the yogic *bandhas*, or locks, such as *Uddiyana bandha* puts pressure on the vagus nerve thereby affecting its function. *Uddiyana bandha* is the belly lock in which the low belly below the navel is drawn in gently towards the spine and slightly up.

Our vocal cords are stimulated by gargling with water or singing loudly, which in turn stimulates the vagus nerve. Warm water or Ayurvedic tea can be used to increase vagal activation. The tone of the vagus nerve can also be aided by moderate or firm foot massage. In addition, splashing your forehead, both eyes, and cheeks in cold water is another option. Laughter improves your mood, strengthens your immune system, and also activates the vagus nerve.

Consuming fiber stimulates vagus nerve impulses to the brain, which facilitate digestive movements and make us feel satiated after meals. High-fiber foods such as dahls, fruits, and dates are excellent choices. The Ayurvedic herbs, being high in fiber, are also helpful options for healthy vagal tone. In addition, preclinical studies have demonstrated that Ayurvedic herbs like turmeric and ginger, as well as bitter herbs like wormwood and gentian, activate the vagus nerve.

Conclusion

The importance of proper management of diet, sleep, stress, and daily routines for the promotion and maintenance of health cannot be overstated. Perhaps this transformation requires a subtle shift in our self-perception. If we recognize our true nature as a boundless organism, we can begin to make the correct choices and thus eat for our microbiome rather than our human cravings.

With our newfound self-awareness, we realize that we are more than just what we eat; rather, we are what we digest and absorb. We can strive to reduce stress because we know it impacts our microbial support system. We appreciate that the benefits of prioritizing sleep extend far beyond an easier morning to support our gut microbiome and immunity. Through this lens of a broader concept of ourselves, we can truly begin to eat, sleep, and establish routines that support the multitudes of microbial supporters within us.

Microbiological insights demonstrate that we are a community, not a discrete organism. In essence, this entire planet is a single, interconnected organism.

Epilogue

We are an interconnected community

Both traditional and modern medical practices acknowledge the importance of the gut in maintaining human health and preventing disease. There is a shared recognition that both health and disease originate primarily in the gastrointestinal tract. The common objective of these distinct medical systems is to transition from states of disease, dysbiosis, and disharmony to health, homeostasis, and harmony. Success entails therapeutically modulating dysbiotic intestinal microbiomes in the direction of health and homeostasis. We should consider ourselves extraordinarily fortunate to have a second opportunity at health in the context of numerous conditions, given that past mistakes can often be rectified by simply modifying our behaviors, routines, and habits. Our gut microbiome is analogous to our own personal bioreactor, so when we change our microbiome, we change ourselves and thus our future.

Ayurveda may represent the original personalized medicine, and genomics-based tools may allow further personalization as a confluence of traditional medicine and modern science emerges. As we gain more knowledge, the various herbal remedies, prebiotics, dietary supplements, or probiotics may be used to increase microbial diversity or modulate the activity of gut microbes to aid in the digestion, bioavailability, and absorption of dietary treatments. In the future, this may be accomplished in an individualized manner using genomic assays to detect and observe intestinal communities as a powerful real-time, global approach to treatment monitoring. Medicinal herbs or prebiotics tailored to the microbiome of the individual patient may one day be used to therapeutically alter the gut microbiome in a targeted and personalized manner.

Including Ayurveda in either the integrative medicine model or as a stand-alone system is of great importance for public health. One reason is that the Western acute care model reigns supreme yet falls short when it comes to the treatment and management of chronic diseases. Ayurveda is markedly effective for the holistic management of chronic diseases, particularly those that are lifestyle-related. One central strength of the Ayurvedic approach is that root causes and early symptoms are identified, whereas the Western medical approach frequently treats the symptoms but not the fundamental cause.

In contrast to allopathic medicine, Ayurvedic treatment emphasizes the necessity to treat the site of imbalance in terms of accumulation and aggravation (the digestive system), the site of overflow of the imbalance (the circulatory system), and the site of relocation of the imbalance if manifestation and diversification have occurred. The wisdom of managing disease early in its development cannot be disregarded. Early detection and management of imbalances are supported by all healthcare disciplines as it is not an 'alternative' notion but one of sound efficiency. Allopathic medicine considers early detection what Ayurveda considers symptoms of *doshic* imbalance relocation, which is considered later stage and more difficult to treat. Ayurveda underscores the earliest phases of disease development and attempts to remedy the imbalance long before later stage symptoms of relocation occur. Despite the direct cost and suffering savings, disease prevention, early detection, and intervention are perceived as less profitable investment strategies by profit-minded corporations, but surely not less profitable to practice for individuals seeking optimal health and longevity.

In addition to the lessons learned from Ayurveda, our microbiomes provide a wealth of information. The microbiome inspires an expanded view of ourselves as a combination of human and bacterial cells and our metabolic characteristics as a functional mixture of human and microbial traits. The number and diversity of the biochemical activities encoded in our microbiomes must be considered important given the sheer size of these populations. Our guts and bodies are figuratively our very own personal bioreactor. We rely so heavily on our gut microbes to digest our dietary plants and perform so many other key functions that we literally cannot live without them. Thus, we should take exceptional care of our gut and digestion with healthy plant-rich diets and daily routines around eating.

The planetary microbes have lived here for 3.5 to 4.2 billion years of the 4.5 billion years of the earth's existence. There is an ancient evolutionary wisdom that can be gained by observing them and viewing the world through a microbial lens. The microbes teach us about life, ourselves, and what it means to be human. Instead of humans being the focal point of existence, a broader microbial perspective positions life in a vaster and more interrelated biochemical context. The microbial world reveals that in community, cooperation, and synergy, great feats are possible. Microbiological insights demonstrate that we are a community, not a discrete organism. In essence, this entire planet is a single, interconnected organism. Consequently, if we are to achieve optimal homeostasis, harmony, and balance in our bodies, communities, and interconnected world, we must approach our environments, bodies, and communities with this philosophy in mind.

www.ingramcontent.com/pod-product-compliance
Lightning Source LLC
Chambersburg PA
CBHW050749150726
48196CB00004B/388